Praise for

25 DAYS

"Despite daily physical and psychological reminders of his sudden cardiac arrest, Drew works hard to deliver an invigorating shock to anyone looking to transform their body! In *25Days* . . . he succeeds!"

—Jeff Ricks, M.D., three-time combat tour veteran,
emergency medicine/mass casualty and trauma expert

"Drew tells it like it is. No double-talk. No pulling punches. No gimmicks or nonsense. The 25Days workout is awesome, the food is great, and the methods for reprogramming your habits are smart. . . . I love it!"

—Kim Lyons, celebrity fitness expert, trainer for NBC's *Biggest Loser*,
IFBB Fitness Pro, and founder of Bionic Body

"Drew is one of the toughest trainers I ever had as a professional athlete. He really knows his stuff, and I am thrilled to see him putting that knowledge in *25Days* for everyone to read!"

—Nazr Mohammed, eighteen-year NBA veteran and world champion

"A good trainer can change your body, but a *great* trainer can change your life. . . . Drew Logan changed my life! *25Days* will change *your* life!"

—Bruno Gunn, actor in *The Hunger Games: Catching Fire*,
Westworld, and *Sons of Anarchy*

"I *love* the message of *25Days*, as well as the simplicity of Drew's programming. Too often we look for quick fixes that don't last, but Drew has created an easy and effective plan for living the best version of yourself!"

—Astrid Swan, celebrity trainer, model, and fitness expert

"A true master can strip away the nonsense and focus on the details that are responsible for success! In *25Days* Drew masterfully guides the reader toward self-discovery and empowerment by making getting in the best shape of your life an attainable goal that can last *forever*! This is more than a valuable tool, it is an indispensable guide!"

—Robert Cabral, 7th degree martial arts master and
founder of Bound Angels Foundation

"There are very few people in our line of work that I consider a peer 100 percent across the board, but Drew Logan is one of them. In *25Days*, Drew shows why he is one of the top elite professionals in the fitness industry by teaching you how working smarter, not just harder, can change your life forever!"

—Bennie Wylie, Jr., coach, Dallas Cowboys, University of Texas,
University of Tennessee, and NBC *Strong* trainer

"Without Drew, I would not have the amazing and fulfilling career I am now enjoying! I fulfilled my potential because Drew gave me the tools to get me where I wanted to go and beyond. If there is anyone capable of changing your life, it's this guy! *25Days* will change your life in ways you never dreamed. . . . *Get this book!*"

—Rick Cosnett, actor in *The Vampire Diaries*, *The Flash*, and *Quantico*

"*25Days* is the ultimate tool for fitness. Drew's practical and precise methods are, all at once, efficient and effective. He's able to break down and demystify the process of getting into your best shape both physically and mentally. His mantra, 'Every day is game day,' will soon be that of many fit and healthy people."

—Jesse L. Martin, actor in *Rent*, *Law & Order*, and *The Flash*

"Drew Logan is a rare force of nature! His *25Days* book is a proven approach to get your mind and body right. If you want an innovative, no-nonsense, creative program to get you great results in little time, read this book!"

—Todd Durkin, trainer, speaker, founder of Fitness Quest 10 gym,
author of *The WOW Book* and *The IMPACT! Body Plan*,
and Under Armour lead fitness advisor

25 DAYS

A PROVEN PROGRAM TO REWIRE YOUR BRAIN, STOP WEIGHT GAIN, AND FINALLY CRUSH THE HABITS YOU HATE—FOREVER

Drew Logan

with Myatt Murphy

G

GALLERY BOOKS

NEW YORK   LONDON   TORONTO   SYDNEY   NEW DELHI

G

Gallery Books
An Imprint of Simon & Schuster, Inc.
1230 Avenue of the Americas
New York, NY 10020

First Gallery Books trade paperback edition September 2018

GALLERY BOOKS and colophon are registered trademarks of Simon & Schuster, Inc.

This publication contains the opinions and ideas of its author. It is sold with the understanding
that the author and publisher are not engaged in rendering health services in the book. The reader
should consult his or her own medical and health providers as appropriate before adopting any of
the suggestions in this book or drawing inferences from it. The author and publisher specifically
disclaim all responsibility for any liability, loss or risk, personal or otherwise, which is incurred as a
consequence, directly or indirectly, of the use and application of any of the contents of this book.

For information about special discounts for bulk purchases, please contact
Simon & Schuster Special Sales at 1-866-506-1949 or business@simonandschuster.com.

The Simon & Schuster Speakers Bureau can bring authors to your live event.
For more information or to book an event, contact the Simon & Schuster Speakers
Bureau at 1-866-248-3049 or visit our website at www.simonspeakers.com.

Interior design by Davina Mock-Maniscalco

Manufactured in the United States of America

10 9 8 7 6 5 4 3 2 1

The Library of Congress has catalogued the North Star Way edition as follows:

Names: Logan, Drew A., author. | Murphy, Myatt, author.
Title: 25Days : a proven program to rewire your brain, stop weight gain, and finally crush the
    habits you hate—forever / by Drew Logan with Myatt Murphy.
Other titles: Twenty-five days
Description: First North Star Way hardcover edition. | New York : North Star Way, 2017.
Identifiers: LCCN 2016047157 | ISBN 9781501162985 (hardback)
Subjects: LCSH: Weight loss—Psychological aspects—Popular works. | Food habits—Psychological
    aspects—Popular works. | Nutrition—Popular works. | BISAC: HEALTH & FITNESS /
    Healthy Living. | HEALTH & FITNESS / Nutrition. | HEALTH & FITNESS / Weight Loss.
Classification: LCC RM222.2 .L554 2017 | DDC 613.2/5—dc23
LC record available at https://lccn.loc.gov/2016047157

ISBN 978-1-5011-6298-5
ISBN 978-1-5011-6300-5 (pbk)
ISBN 978-1-5011-6299-2 (ebook)

My name is Drew Logan, and I'm forty-two years old. I work twelve-hour days and need a cardiac therapy dog 24-7 that smells my hormones to alert me whenever I'm stressed out. I've been *dead* three times and have a garage door opener inside my chest. I'm also in the best shape of my life, despite what you've just read, because my brain no longer holds me back from being my best self.

That's *my* story.

So, do you know what type of body your brain may be keeping from you?

Contents

Is Your Life Worth Twenty-five Days?

Why twenty-five days? you ask. Let's just say I'm partial to numbers that finally work in my favor.

If you've ever heard of the notion that death always comes in threes, I can personally vouch for that. In my case, death came three times for me in the same night. But instead of losing my life, the experience changed it, affecting the way I would view health and fitness from that day forward.

It was October 4, 2004, midway through my twenty-one-year career in fitness and nutrition, when, while I was seated at the computer, my heart—

simply—

stopped—

beating.

Thirty seconds later, I recovered on my own, only to have my heart fail again minutes later. I had no pulse. I wasn't breathing. I was officially dead for the second time for about six minutes before being revived by a paramedic, who plunged a big needle full of epinephrine into my heart and defibrillated me three times.

My heart was beating, but I had been without oxygen to my brain to the point where my lungs had already shut down. I had a pulse but no lung activity, so they hooked me up to a ventilator and rushed me to the hospital. That's where my heart quit on me a third and final time. It took a minimum of ten defibrillations to bring me back to life before I fell into a coma for three days. But that night, I made the history books in a way I wouldn't wish on anyone.

I died three times in three hours and became the world's only known medical case to survive three consecutive sudden cardiac arrests (SCA) without any kind of implanted defibrillator.

When I woke up, I began to pull out all of my intravenous tubes because I didn't understand where I was—all I knew was that I wanted to get out of there. They sedated me and removed me from life support, but I had no short-term memory. I didn't know who my parents were, or my girlfriend. You could tell me something, and ninety seconds later, I wouldn't know what you were talking about. But it wasn't amnesia. It was simply the inability to retain anything. In fact, to this day, I have a blank space in my brain and can't recall anything from October 4 until Thanksgiving—two months of my life are still missing from my memory.

After enduring a week's worth of tests and having a cardio defibrillator device implanted in my chest, I was sent home with no real answers. The medical community was surprised that I had survived and shocked that it had found nothing wrong with my heart or any evidence of damage. The only two things doctors were certain about was that a "random" electrical malfunction—most likely stress—had caused my SCAs and that my being in shape and living a healthy lifestyle were behind the fact that I was still alive.

Even though I left the hospital with what seemed to be a normal working brain, I knew something wasn't quite right. Due to the lack of oxygen flow to my brain during my SCAs, I couldn't stay focused and even found myself suffering from clinical depression. It wouldn't be until much later, after being diagnosed by Jeff Ricks, MD, one of the world's foremost experts on mass trauma management, that I would discover I had battled what is known medically as mild brain trauma. But at that moment, I just knew that the way my brain was working was not working for me.

Up until my incident, I had been working as a personal trainer for ten years and had been working extensively with NFL and NBA athletes in their off-seasons. During that time, I trained both myself and my clients using very strict routines: carefully planned workouts designed to prevent plateaus by gradually changing the intensity, specificity, and volume over the course of twelve to twenty weeks. The diets I relied on were even more complicated, involving three separate twelve- to twenty-week phases.

I was a measurer, a calorie counter, and focused on every single nutrient level in every single food. I even wore a watch and set alarms to remind myself to eat at exact times, just to try to capitalize on my body's hormonal functions around whatever stimulus I was getting by eating a particular food. If all that sounds confusing, trust me, it was. In fact, it was nauseating.

But after my SCAs, I was suddenly someone who had to monitor his stress, so it was unhealthy for me to follow complex and frustrating programs anymore. I was also still someone who couldn't remember what he had just done minutes before. Sometimes my watch would go off, and I wouldn't know what meal I was on. Sometimes I wouldn't even know what day it was. It was unbearable and undoable, which was why I decided to stop everything I was trying to do and simplify it. I had to work around my brain to keep my body from falling apart.

Instead of trying to focus on exercise and diet programs lasting twelve to twenty weeks, I started focusing on one meal at a time. One snack at a time. One workout at a time. And for each time I ate healthy or finished a workout, I gave myself a grade of 100 percent. At the end of the day, I would sit down and go over everything I had done—even if I didn't remember doing half of what was on my list. If I managed to do everything and I scored 100 percent on every meal, snack, and workout, I considered myself successful.

And the next day, I would do it again. And the day after that.

At the end of the week, I added up my total score to see how successful I had been for five days straight. After five consecutive blocks of five days, I added up my score again, just to have a sense of the past month. Eventually, as my short-term memory slowly returned and my depression lifted, within months, I was a changed man—both physically and mentally. I was imminently aware that something felt better about the program compared with methods I had used in the past.

Beyond getting back into incredible shape, the first thing I noticed was how calm I became. I was no longer as worried about how my meals were balanced, and I stopped weighing and measuring everything. Instead, I took an eyeball approach with all my servings. I knew I was still eating healthy, but I took a very general preventive health approach to my diet, instead of the very strict, hard-line approach I had been used to following.

I also noticed that I was no longer *that* person who was hard to go out to eat with, so my friends no longer had to kill themselves trying to find restaurants that could accommodate my crazy dietary habits. Suddenly I could eat anywhere. I accepted that every meal wouldn't be perfect but so long as I ate certain foods, everything would be all right.

I returned to work as a top trainer three months after my incident and started using 25Days with clients immediately. But to be honest, I didn't start them on it because of the amazing results I had seen in myself; I did it because it was the only way I could keep track of their programs! I had them carry journals and grade themselves at every meal, snack, and day I wasn't training them, so I always knew exactly what to do and where they had slipped along the way.

It made my training job easier and made their outcomes more enjoyable for them by streamlining my approach to diet and exercise into a twenty-five-day block of time. By having them focus on what *really* mattered to get results, and asking them to grade themselves each day, it left my clients feeling equally relaxed and as if they were kicking life in the ass each and every day. And then an interesting thing happened.

Before my SCAs, I had always had a great success rate with all my clients in getting them to get onto the difficult-to-manage nutrition programs I was suggesting. But even though I had a really high success rate, it wasn't maintainable *practically* in a real-world situation. Suddenly my clients weren't just hitting their fitness and weight loss goals faster and more often, they were making positive changes within other facets of their lives—and feeling like a success every step of the way.

So . . . Is Your Life Worth Twenty-five Days?

For me, 25Days didn't start as a choice—it began as something I needed to do to overcome an obstacle.

I can't eliminate my obstacle. I see it every day when I step out of the shower and notice the scar on my chest. I'm reminded whenever I look down at Lucky, my heart therapy service dog who works with me twenty-four hours a day. I'm aware of it each time I offer him my palm to lick to make sure I'm doing okay—and any time he gets me out of harm's way if he senses my cortisol levels going through the roof unexpectedly.

No, I can't eliminate my obstacle, but I have no fear of it anymore. I've become stronger than my obstacle—and so can you. So tell me, what's your obstacle?

I know you have one, or you wouldn't be reading this. We all have some kind of barrier to becoming the best version of ourselves. And for many, that obstacle is usually doubt or fear of failure. Either way, it makes them feel that they can never be successful.

So I challenge you with this: Is your life worth twenty-five days?

Is the effort of putting in just twenty-five days too much to risk to eliminate that obstacle for the rest of your life?

If, after twenty-five days, you begin to uncover a way to be consistently healthy so you can live a life of full potential, then isn't it worth it to try doing away with that obstacle? I want you to have the best life possible, and the way to do that is through the same commonsense, straightforward, no-nonsense approach that saved me and has been successful with all of my clients. That's what the 25Days program is really all about. That said, take a deep breath. Now blow it out. If you've failed every other time in your life or you've never tried for fear of failing, I want you to relax. This will be the time you succeed. This is the way to be able to stay healthy for the rest of your life. This is the way to rewire your brain to make it effortless to make the choices necessary to live the life you deserve.

This is so much easier than you think it is. Just give me twenty-five days to show you.

part one

WHY TWENTY-FIVE DAYS? BLAME YOUR BRAIN!

chapter one

Train Your Brain to Stop the Gain

I n my profession, I don't have a lot of time to create results with people, and there is nobody committed like the recently converted. That's why the thing I've probably said more than anything else to my clients over the last twenty-two years is this:

> **"I can change your body faster than you can learn why it's changing—if you just do exactly what I ask of you."**

All of my clients always know they're more than welcome to learn every detail behind why they're succeeding. But when asked if they want to change first and understand why later—or understand how it all works before they begin their lifelong transformation—well, let's just say it's pretty obvious that most (if not all) prefer their results now and the reasons why much later on.

Maybe that's you. And if it is, I get that. And if so, then don't worry: you'll be starting sooner than you think. But before you begin 25Days, whether you love or hate details, I need you to know the truth about fitness, what's been holding you back from reaching your goals, and how you're going to rewire your brain to finally stop the gain.

The Cram-and-Purge Problem

When it comes to fitness, weight loss, and living a healthier lifestyle, have you ever asked yourself, "***Why*** am I doing the same things over and over again—and never seeming to succeed?"

Here's the answer: the problem might never have been that you weren't doing the right things or that you hadn't done the right things for a long enough period of time. It's just that you were putting your hopes in something that had an expiration date on it.

I've never liked the idea of "Lose five pounds in five days!" or "Get skinny for summer!" or any other end goal. In my mind, that's a very nonsensical way to approach fitness because it teaches you to reach a set objective, whether it's hitting a certain number on the scale or feeling good about fitting into your summer jeans. And then, once you've reached that goal, guess what? You think you're suddenly fixed.

My problem with that cram-and-purge mentality is that it feeds into something we're taught as early as grade school. When we were young, the game plan was always the same: study everything possible, take a test, get the grade—and then flush out all that information as if it had never existed. It was all about *cramming* in what you need to know and *purging* it when it was over.

I'm sure if I asked you to memorize all fifty-two words of the preamble to the US Constitution, you could cram it into your brain and recite it verbatim in an hour, but I'll bet you wouldn't remember it word for word the next day. Why? Because the cram-and-purge method is only a temporary solution. It's a neurological strategy used to teach a learned action in response to achieving some sort of goal or deadline.

Even when we're through with school, that cram-and-purge mentality stays with us. Think about it: every business in the world has some daily, weekly, monthly, or yearly goal or deadline that must be reached by a particular time. No matter what you do for a living—whether you're a CEO or a stay-at-home mom—there's no escaping the pressure of deadlines and goals.

Health, diet, and fitness aren't any different in how people commonly approach them. For many (and I'll be willing to bet that's you), the solution to becoming leaner and healthier has always been to rely on some form of cram-and-purge. And, depending on how well that approach worked for you in the past, it may secretly be behind why you've always had difficulty losing weight—no matter how hard you've tried.

For many, cramming and purging can be a stressful experience, because of the pressure, the fear of failing, or both. It's a challenge that instantly comes with a negative connotation, which is why many people either avoid most weight loss programs or quit before they see results.

For those who manage to stick it out and reach their goals, odds are, that's it. Because once they reach their target weight, or whatever their goal was, a few days later they find themselves gradually going right back to their old habits. All of the weight lost comes right back—plus a little more. Sadly, everything crammed and purged never turns into a lifestyle; it just becomes discarded until the next bikini season or class reunion.

Another major flaw with cram and purge is that you feel successful only at the "end" of the journey—and never during the journey itself. In other words, with most diet plans you always have to wait until it's over until you're allowed to feel like a winner.

A lot of my female clients tend to be extremely dedicated to the cause. Once they're ready to lose weight, most will go nauseatingly hard with crazy motivation and focus, which is a wonderful thing. But the problem is that most have only an end result in mind.

One of my most successful clients was an amazing woman who was having trouble losing her baby weight. Throughout her early twenties, she had been a runner, played field hockey, and participated in a variety of activities. But in her late twenties, two years after having her first child, she still couldn't get rid of sixty pounds.

When she came to me, she was unhappy because she wasn't operating at her potential and wasn't exactly where she wanted to be. All she could focus on was the sixty pounds she needed to lose, instead of celebrating the fact that she did everything right that first day when it came to exercising and eating right.

There's a lot of weight lifted from your mind when you understand that you can be successful day in and day out. When you remove all doubt, it just makes it that much easier to keep doing what you're doing. I got her to understand that she didn't need to worry about losing sixty pounds; all she needed to do was succeed today.

And then tomorrow.

And the day after that.

She had to focus only on the day at hand, knowing that each day was linked to a greater plan. I showed her how to use each day to feel confident that she was always moving steadily in the right direction. Those sixty pounds are long gone now—and have stayed off, by the way—because they stopped being a goal. Instead, they simply became the end result of living and maintaining a healthy 25Days lifestyle.

Are you going to make that happen for yourself in twenty-five days? Because most people's fitness goals aim high, probably not. But you'll be in much better shape in twenty-five days than you were before. And you'll be in even better shape twenty-five days after that. More important, you'll be throwing away the cram-and-purge mind-set that's always failed you, using a program you'll never want to discard—and will want to use for life.

The Neurological Pattern Predicament

As a highly educated strength coach, certified fitness trainer, and specialist in performance nutrition, I'm considered an expert in understanding exactly how the body works. But when I began using 25Days myself and with my clients, what I couldn't comprehend was why it made getting into and staying in great shape so easy to do. Why, even after my clients reached their fitness and weight loss goals, they found it just as effortless as I had to turn the program into a lifestyle.

What I'd come to discover is that 25Days had **essentially *rewired our brains in a way that made it easier to lead and stick with a healthier lifestyle.***

That realization began after meeting with medical experts to tackle the mild brain trauma that had resulted from my SCAs. As I started working with doctors to pull apart and address what was going on inside my brain, I happened to discuss the program I had designed to keep myself on track—and my doctor smiled. What I quickly came to discover is that my program had indirectly created positive behaviors that had replaced the negative behaviors that had been partially responsible for almost killing me.

It comes down to this: even though people love to use the phrase "We are all creatures of habit," it's what's behind our repeated behaviors that's much more important to understand. We're all driven by a particular set of neurological patterns—patterns we build over time that imprint onto our brains. Whenever you crave or repeat a behavior, whether it's something good or bad for you, there's a neurological pattern causing that action or behavior, whether you're conscious of it or not.

In fact, according to the Society for Personality and Social Psychology,* roughly 40 percent of the activities you do throughout the day are automatic responses you're often not even aware you're doing. Think about that: almost half of your day is spent unconsciously repeating the same behaviors over and over again, due to having certain neurological patterns in place. And if those behaviors are negative, you're spending almost half your day unconsciously doing things that are preventing you from reaching your full potential.

How do those neurological patterns get there in the first place? They commonly form around the release of either hormones (signaling molecules produced by the endocrine glands that travel through the bloodstream) or neurotransmitters (chemicals that transmit messages from one brain cell to another). For example, whenever we do something that causes the brain to release any of the so-called happy chemicals—such as endorphins, serotonin, oxytocin, or dopamine, we feel good—but the feeling doesn't last. Once that rush is over, we want more of it, which is how we start carving out an unhealthy neurological pattern.

We may repeat behaviors initially for the hormonal or neurotransmitter response we get from them, but eventually, it's the repetition that

---

*Wendy Wood, "Habits in Everyday Life: How to Form Good Habits and Change Bad Ones" (poster session, American Psychological Association's 122nd Annual Convention, Washington, DC, August 7, 2014).

becomes the problem. According to research from University College London,[*] it can take 15 to 254 days to form a new neurological pattern, with the average being just 66 days.

The good news: there is a three-step process to overwrite undesirable neurological patterns and replace them with healthier patterns:

1. The first step is through **disrupting existing behaviors caused by unhealthy neurological patterns** to "make space," if you will, for a new and healthier neurological pattern to form.

2. The second step is through **simple repetition**: the more consistently you repeat a behavior, the faster you'll build a neurological pattern around it.

3. The crucial third step is **making sure there are cues that help trigger the new neurological pattern.**

What I found out quickly was that my program was automatically making this three-step process take place. In addition to being an easier method for building lean muscle and boosting metabolism, I had been triggering positive brain chemical responses and preventing negative ones through the right combination of meals, workouts, and rewards. I had essentially created a program that naturally made it easier to stay on track by simply giving the brain enough stimuli and time to form new, healthier neurological patterns—in as little as twenty-five days.

DREW LOGAN

[*]Phillippa Lally et al., "How Are Habits Formed: Modelling Habit Formation in the Real World," *European Journal of Social Psychology* 40, no. 6 (2010): 998–1009.

chapter two

Breaking the Brain Barrier

F itness doesn't have to be complex—it's just been made to seem that way. The truth is this: I could sew this whole thing up on one page and even write it in crayon: I want you to scare your fat cells and make your muscle cells excited enough to change.

That's it.

Thank you very much, and have a great day.

Point being, if you eat and do the right things, your body will respond in kind exactly as you want it to by becoming leaner, healthier, and fitter. But the main reason most people aren't leaner, healthier, and fitter isn't because they don't know *what* to do. It's that they don't know how to forge the positive neurological patterns that can make doing all of those necessary things an easier, unconscious part of their daily routine.

The Dope on Dopamine

To understand the basics of why 25Days is so effective at retraining your brain to switch out old neurological patterns for new, healthier ones, you need to understand the power and importance of dopamine.

Dopamine is the neurotransmitter you have to thank for controlling the brain's pleasure and reward centers. It's the biochemical that gets released and gives you pleasure whenever you do something rewarding, which makes you more likely to repeat that behavior again.

Smoking, drinking alcohol, and eating sugar-laden or high-fat foods all trigger the release of dopamine, which is the main reason so many people have a hard time curbing or stepping away from certain bad-for-you vices. In fact, what many interpret as an addiction can often be a simple neurological pattern built by the release of dopamine in the nucleus accumbens, the reward center of the brain.

Conversely, there are certain situational stimuli that can bring about a negative brain chemical response. For example, lack of sleep and high stress are just two of the things that can trigger a dopamine release, even though both situations are harmful to your body. Have you ever known someone whose life is always in a state of chaos? The person who always seems to find himself or herself in a whirlwind of problems? It might be that he or she is either creating or following the drama, due to being addicted to the dopamine response typically associated with it.

But dopamine isn't a one-trick pony. What a lot of people fail to remember is that it is meant to be a reward for a job well done. You get a dopamine response whenever you finish a task, receive a promotion, hit a home run, or discover that perfectly sized pair of shoes you've always wanted on sale. It's what gives you that confident feeling from having accomplished something.

When I started using 25Days, it didn't have a name—but it was always about *today*. I didn't want clients thinking about how many pounds they had to lose or which numbers they wanted to raise or lower before their next doctor's visit. All I wanted them to do was win today. And then tomorrow. And soon, before they realized it, they'd made the right neurological changes that allowed them to succeed at staying in shape and healthy for the rest of their lives.

What I didn't realize at first was how my program was manipulating my clients' dopamine levels in a way that made it much easier for them to form new, healthy neurological patterns. But once I finally made that connection, I discovered the power behind limiting the negative stimuli that cause a dopamine response while simultaneously stimulating a dopamine response around positive fitness and health-related behaviors. That's why I've spent the last twelve years fine-tuning a diet and exercise program that controls and magnifies that reward response to help form healthy neurological patterns in an average of just twenty-five days.

From Grades to Goals

Way back when, you set a series of neurological patterns in place that are responsible for making you the type of person you are right now: unhappy with your unhealthy behaviors and dissatisfied with the shape you're in.

The fact is, most people desire to be fit, and they *basically* know what they need to do to make that happen, but the sensation of looking forward to eating healthier and exercising feels foreign to many. Maybe enjoying the journey toward getting in shape seems as strange to you as intentionally getting out of shape seems to me—it just doesn't compute. I get it, but what if you could change that?

The way 25Days works is simple:

+ Each day, you'll eat three meals and one to two snacks. Every meal or snack has to contain what I like to call Put-Ins. These Put-Ins are equally simple: you'll eat a certain amount of protein, healthy fats, low-glycemic fibrous carbohydrates, and a glass of water. If you get everything in each meal or snack, you earn 20 percent or 25 percent (depending on how many times you ate that day). Eat all of your meals and snacks the right way, and your grade is 100 percent.

+ Each day, you'll also be asked to do some form of workout. If you finish your workout, your total grade is 100 percent.

+ Once you have both numbers, you'll add them together to get your average grade—and that's it.

+ You'll tally up your grade every night for twenty-five days. You'll also average out your grade every five days and then take a final average of all twenty-five days at the end to receive a final grade.

✦ Finally, you'll cut out certain activities and foods that are not only unhealthy for your body but also unhealthy for your brain.

That daily grade is the backbone of 25Days. My program lets you feel successful every day and every single meal. Each grade gives you that constant positive affirmation that you're on the right track, like mile markers along a road letting you know that you're traveling in the right direction. But that's not what makes the grading system special.

Being able to access instantly how well you've eaten and exercised each day, and seeing, through your grade, how successful you were at finishing a task, triggers an immediate dopamine release response that makes you feel good. So at the end of the day, you'll have elicited a powerful dopamine response—a reward for a job well done—that's tied directly to those positive behaviors. Those consistent dopamine responses will help keep you on course long enough to carve out new, healthier neurological patterns.

You see, every time you elicit that dopamine response, it evokes a loud and pronounced awareness, if you will, that something is different, starting on Day 1. And from that feeling of something "being different" every single day, your mind begins to create neurological patterns around that loud and pronounced activity. It makes your brain begin to associate what you're undertaking with 25Days as positive. It makes it believe that eating better and exercising each day are not only a good thing but also something that you should and need to continue.

If you're that person I mentioned earlier—the one who doesn't look forward to getting fit—I want you to know that by trying 25Days, you'll be making a loud and pronounced wake-up call to your brain. I want you to know you will win right from Day 1. And soon, before you know it, you'll have made the neurological changes that will allow you to succeed at this for the rest of your life. If you're fed up with trying to *wrap* your head around getting in shape, 25Days will give you the power to *rewire* your brain to get into your best shape ever.

The 85 Percent Promise

As I began to change the neurological patterns in my clients, I started to notice something about 25Days that I continue to see today. Anyone I have ever trained, and anyone I have ever known, has always reached his or her goals by putting in just 85 percent. That's why, ideally, I want you to get through 25Days with a final grade of 85 percent or above.

Don't get me wrong. I'd be thrilled to see you hit 100 percent right out of the gate, but if you don't, that doesn't mean you didn't win. The truth is, some days you're the bear—and some days, the bear eats you.

That's the beauty of 25Days. Each day is a stand-alone and not your entire life. You don't have to be perfect with your diet and exercise every single day, because *no one* is perfect. Once you know and embrace that fact, it takes a huge burden off the pressure of trying to reach your health and fitness goals.

There's a statement I make to all of my clients (and it's one that I make quite often): *it matters less what you're doing with specificity than it matters what you're doing consistently.*

I don't know any special diet secret that someone else doesn't know. I don't know any special exercise routine that's better than the rest. And, by the way, if anyone else tells you he or she does, that person is lying. **The reality is, I've put everything your brain and body needs into a structure that gives you the feeling of being a success every single day**—and that's important.

Because when you feel that way at the end of the day, you'll wake up the next day and want to do it again. And pretty soon, you'll find yourself wanting to experience that feeling all the time. Not only that, but you'll also discover you've unconsciously rewired your brain in a way that makes sticking with a healthier lifestyle from that point forward effortless and more enjoyable.

In my career, I've used a lot of great programs that have worked successfully, but I've had the most long-term success with this method. Even when I've tried to step away from 25Days with certain clients, they haven't been nearly as successful as the ones who have used this tried-and-true grading system.

What I want you to know is this: you don't have to wait until the seventieth day of your XYZ twelve-week program to start feeling good about yourself. You can do it today—and you will be a success today. And you can be a success tomorrow.

chapter three

Why 25Days Is All It Takes

When I first created 25Days for myself, my goal was simply to make it easier to get a handle on my diet and exercise. I just needed something that would tell me what to do and make me feel confident that I was doing exactly what needed to be accomplished.

Even with my clients, I find that no matter who I train—from celebrities and CEOs to multisport athletes and multikid moms—every client is either a *need-to-do-now* type of person or a *need-to-know-first* kind of person. Either mentality works with 25Days.

If you're a **need-to-do-now** type—the kind of person who couldn't care less about why something works and just wants to get into the driver's seat and take 25Days around the block immediately, I'm going to give you the freedom to do exactly that. But if you're a **need-to-know-first** person who won't listen to diet and exercise advice until you know all the ins and outs about what they're being asked to do it, and why, then I respect that too. That's why this book is divided into two separate sections.

25Days: Simplified or Magnified—You Decide!

The problem with a lot of lifestyle and diet books is that sometimes many science-minded experts (myself included) like to overthink the process. I'll admit it: I love to talk about the research and scientific data regarding exercise and diet. But I also know that those I serve don't always need to understand things at an expert level to get the results they're seeking.

That's why most of the chapters from this point forward are divided into two sections: **25Days Simplified** and **25Days Magnified**!

If you're the **need-to-do-now** type, you can skip whole portions of this book and jump feetfirst into 25Days. You'll start each chapter and read up until you come to **25Days Simplified**. Once there, you'll learn the real bedrock on what to do, without my getting into too much detail or your ever feeling overwhelmed wondering *why* you're doing it. Finish that portion, and you can move on to the next chapter.

If you're the **need-to-know-first** type, I have you covered as well. Just read 25Days from cover to cover as you would any other book. Where relevant, you'll find more information in the **25Days Magnified** sections. There I'll teach you about what's behind certain key 25Days strategies as you learn about them. To give you a taste of how it works:

The 25Days Program *Simplified*!

Aesthetics aside—I don't want to see how many pounds or belt sizes you hope to lose—grab a piece of paper and write down five things about yourself you would love to change over the next twenty-five days.

If you're a **need-to-do-now** type, you're done! Put away that sheet for the next twenty-five days. If you're ready to start and have no interest—for now—in learning why I asked you to write down those five things or about how I adapted 25Days to be even more efficient at evoking certain brain chemical responses, just turn to the next chapter.

But if you're curious and you're also wondering what other additional benefits 25Days may offer beyond forging new, healthier neurological patterns, then you're ready for . . .

The 25Days Program *Magnified*!

Perhaps you think the only thing that makes 25Days different is a grading system that helps you change your brain. But there's much more going on behind the scenes. Beyond the basics, the program relies on three fundamental principles to help elicit dopamine in larger doses—and at the right moments—to make forming new, healthier neurological patterns an easier and much faster process: triggers, techniques, and timing.

1. TRIGGERS

The cornerstone of 25Days uses the release of dopamine to help rewire your brain, but it's not as simple as that. The program is designed in such a way that you'll release your two largest bursts of dopamine in the morning (after your workout) and after receiving your grade at the end of the day. By burning the candle at both ends, 25Days helps to trigger a dopamine-and-endorphin (a brain hormone that relieves pain) response from physical exertion and a dopamine response from the accomplishment of a job well done, which produces a very strong psychological effect.

These are the two positive behaviors I want your brain to start associating as the primary drivers of dopamine, so it can immediately begin building positive neurological patterns around regular exercise and eating right. The trick is, the longer you can delay the release of dopamine throughout the day, the more intense a dopamine release you'll feel at the end of the day when you receive your grade.

That's why it is equally important to minimize other dopamine triggers—such as stress, lack of sleep, and even certain foods—during your day. If you consistently experience little bursts of dopamine all day long from other triggers, it can minimize the amount of that second burst, making it less effective at helping you build a neurological pattern around positive behaviors.

25Days takes that into account by reducing a variety of other daily dopamine triggers, so you always receive the greatest brain-changing surge of dopamine at the end of the day. In addition to reducing stress and promoting sleep, the diet itself is rich in foods that are high in tyrosine, the main building block of dopamine. Examples include almonds, avocados, chicken, eggs, and beef.

2. TECHNIQUES

There are many ways to exercise, but not every method is ideal if you're trying to accomplish brain change. Certain high-intensity techniques—or simply exercising too long—can overtax the central nervous system and lead to *overtraining*.* Push yourself too hard and for too long, and you can also lower your levels of certain important neurotransmitters such as glutamine (an amino acid essential for preventing your body from breaking down muscle tissue for energy) and 5-hydroxytryptophan, or 5-HTP (an amino acid shown to curb appetite and lead to weight loss). What sets 25Days apart is that it alternates between two unique types of workout techniques that together provide the right amount of stimulation to build lean muscle and burn fat, while offering just enough time in between for your muscles and central nervous system to heal and recover.

Another reason why 25Days has been so successful for my clients and me is in its balance. Many people fail to lose weight on other programs because they rely too much on either exercise or diet. In fact, I've had some clients ask, "Which portion makes it so efficient? Is it 80/20 diet versus exercise or 70/30 exercise over diet?"

My answer is always the same: they are equally important parts of a total successful program. But it's not a 50/50 split—it's a 100/100 effort. Why do I say that? Because if you tell clients that a program is 50/50, then they sometimes don't give their all to each component. What I need you to understand is that both your diet and your exercise work in concert with each other on 25Days. You're going to get the best results only by doing them both, because you can't out-train a bad diet—and you can't out-eat a weak body. It takes 100 percent attention to both, which is why 25Days focuses on diet and exercise equally.

3. TIMING

The third factor that most people never consider is the impact of *when* they decide to eat or exercise. Even though some may understand the importance of spacing out their meals every few hours or not eating carbohydrates after a certain time of the evening, being a little stricter—and more consistent—when it comes to when you eat and when you sweat

---

*Jeffrey B. Kreher and Jennifer B. Schwartz, "Overtraining Syndrome: A Practical Guide," *Sports Health* 4, no. 2 (2012): 128–38, doi:10.1177/1941738111434406.

plays an equally important part in how quickly it takes to rewire your brain.

25Days relies on having you stick to an exact schedule of when you eat and exercise for your brain's sake. By performing certain healthy behaviors at the same time every day, it teaches your body to begin anticipating those behaviors, which makes it much easier to develop a neurological pattern around them.

The program also takes into account when you're most likely to give yourself too much slack. How so? The typical workweek is five days, Monday through Friday. That's also generally the only time people live according to a routine. It also means that for most people, their Saturdays and Sundays tend to become free-for-alls on everything, from what we eat and how we sleep to whether we exercise or not.

Those two days become the excuse for us to overeat, drink too much, and do little to absolutely nothing when it comes to physical activity. That's why 25Days is divided into five-day blocks of time—not a seven-days-a-week schedule. That way, regardless of what day it is on the calendar, you're sure to stick to the program and see the most results.

The 25Days Difference

The additional benefits that my program brings to the table go far beyond rewiring your brain in as little as twenty-five days. It does everything that most diet and weight loss programs never do—and even works with you, in case you can't give up what you're currently doing.

25Days Gives You Instant Feedback

Getting a grade each day isn't just about dopamine—it's also an important number that instantly lets you know where you stand. Having an immediate sense of how you're doing today—and how you did every day before that—is what many programs lack, but it's what dieters need to stay motivated and moving forward.

One of the biggest benefits of the 25Days grading system is that it lets you look back at your previous day's efforts and know instantly that you're doing all of the right things and are on the proper path—so that you're less likely to take a detour due to doubt. Think of those past grades as your "**Comfort Compass**."

25Days Keeps You in the Process

The intrinsic value of 25Days is that it keeps your mind in a state of conscious awareness. You see, most people's approach to a healthy lifestyle—especially when it comes to their nutrition—is reactionary, not *proactive*. It's almost done unconsciously. For example, if I walked up to you on the street at eight in the morning and asked what you planned on having for dinner two nights from now, odds are you wouldn't have any idea.

The way 25Days is designed, what you eat and what you need to do exercisewise are always placed in the front of your mind. It's a conscious, proactive program that keeps you in the moment because you're always thinking about each meal and each workout. You're left with no choice but to stay conscious of what you're doing throughout the day, which brings about a constant sense of instant accountability.

25Days Offers More Guidance and Less Guilt

Everyone makes mistakes, and no one's perfect. There will be days when you'll achieve a grade of 85 percent or higher, and there might be days when you don't. You might not be ready for certain exercises this time around, and you might experience moments of weakness when you grab a slice of pizza instead of a piece of fresh grilled fish.

Unlike other lifestyle books that typically offer either negative reinforcement for screwing up or no advice at all, 25Days anticipates the mistakes many people make. The thing to remember is that I've used 25Days myself and with my clients for over a decade, so I know all of the bumps in the road that people sometimes encounter.

That's why throughout the book at key locations, you'll find a series of "*If-Then*" statements to guide you in the event of any mood swings, insulin spikes, cravings, or temporary hormonal/brain chemical changes that may occur if you stumble along the way. In other words, you'll know exactly what to expect—in many cases *before* it even happens—so that you can make the necessary adjustments to get back on track.

25Days Prevents the Dreaded Weight-ing Room Gloom

I always tell clients, "You're not going to get in shape *today*, but you're going to get in shape after a consistent number of successful todays." That's why my biggest problem with most programs that actually work has always been this: the only two times you truly feel successful is when you see those "instant results" at the very beginning, and if—and that's a big *if*—you've reached your target goal.

The problem is that the distance between the two can leave you always feeling as if you're in limbo, with no sense of when you might reach your goal. With no finish line in sight, most people quit. But with 25Days, you're always less than a day away from your next finish line. You never feel as if you're in the middle of a massive chunk of time—because your absolute attention always remains on today, and not on the tomorrow that you think will never come.

25Days Keeps You from Throwing It All Away

In a traditional weight loss program, even though you may be warned about having harder days than others, you're typically expected to stay the path. So when you mess up one day along the way, it becomes that much easier to talk yourself into stopping the entire process to try again another time. Even on a micro level, when was the last time you found yourself eating more than you should at a meal, and then used that slipup as an excuse to blow the entire day?

Imagine failing a school quiz a few weeks into a class. Would you quit? Would you run to the principal and ask that they pull you out? Of course not. The fact of the matter is, even if you made a few mistakes that cost you a good grade, you'd still remain in the class—if you wanted to progress to the next level. You'd pay the penalty, but you'd stick it out. 25Days doesn't prevent you from creating an excuse to start over—because it doesn't allow you to start over.

With 25Days, the tendency to "throw it all away" never occurs because there's always a way to salvage the day if you eat smarter and exercise right. All that matters is how you eat at that *next* meal or the *next* time you exercise—your success is never stopped by a single moment of weakness. With 25Days, the good days can easily outweigh the bad, bringing you right back in the direction of your goals.

25Days Moves with You–It Doesn't Leave You Behind

A lot of exercise plans have expectations from week to week. So when you don't have the energy to eat even cleaner or master certain exercises at the time you're supposed to, that can leave you feeling like a failure. They don't adjust with you—they expect you to adjust to them.

25Days progresses at your body's natural pace. Maybe you're the type who quickly moves through a program and needs to modify it immediately because you get stronger, fitter, and more conditioned at a faster pace. Or maybe your body likes to take its time to adjust. Either way, the program is designed around completion, not changing how much weight you're using or expecting you to be strong enough to do certain exercises that might not be in your wheelhouse just yet.

It's not even about how hard you perform or how much you do (although it's nice to have those little checks and balances as you time your workouts). Will there will be moments when you realize you're starting to complete your workouts in less time? Yes. But the reality is that some days you're going to be more tired than on other days. I don't even care if you phone it in some days and it takes you twice as long to complete a workout. That's fine, so long as you find the energy to complete it. That's all that matters.

25Days Works with the Workouts You Do Already

I've met people from all walks of life—dancers, track stars, swimmers, bodybuilders, CrossFitters, runners, and athletes of every shape and size—and everybody thinks that his or her way of working out is the only way. The reality is, none of that is true. There is no one perfect exercise or one perfect workout.

Ready for some more truth? And if you've ever heard a celeb trainer tell you that "their plan" is the best and only plan, know this: it's simply not true. If what you're being told isn't a boldfaced lie or misrepresentation, then it's a miseducation and misunderstanding of the way the body works and what is most beneficial for your body.

I understand how life works. Maybe you already have a particular workout regimen in place, and you're not willing to give it up quite yet. 25Days won't stop you from what may be working for you; nor does it keep you from doing what you love. It's designed only to change the neurological patterns that may be holding you back.

The workouts in 25Days were created to make exercising excuse-proof if you don't have access to equipment. It's also scalable, so you can move it up or down to match your current fitness level. It's a workout that I use with my clients because I can do it anywhere.

That being said, if this isn't the type of workout you want to do, or you love what you're already doing, that's fine. The heart of 25Days isn't about the workouts or the diet—it's in the plan. As long as you are using a workout that meets the criteria I need you to do each day (I'll explain those rules later on), you can use whatever you wish. I can guarantee that your outcome with those routines will be even better doing them the 25Days way.

WEIGHT ASIDE, WHAT DO YOU *REALLY* NEED TO CHANGE IN TWENTY-FIVE DAYS?

It doesn't take a lot of deep soul diving to come up with what you want to change aesthetically. I'll be honest: even fit people step out of the shower, look at themselves, and say, "I'd like to change that!" That's why I stressed at the start of this chapter to put aside your weight and do a true evaluation of yourself before beginning the program. I want you to begin identifying those things outside of your gut and butt that need equal attention.

The reasons I do this with clients are threefold. One, I want you to recognize that there are other things happening in your life that are just as important—if not more important—than merely looking better in the mirror or fitting into a certain dress size. Things that you're probably ignoring or writing off as something else—things you will begin to notice drastically improve each time you try 25Days.

Two, getting you to write down these things also provides multiple forms of motivation. Each one is its own separate motivator. So when you find yourself needing to dig deep during 25Days, suddenly you have five other reasons to stick with the program, instead of just staying the course to improve what you see on the outside.

Finally, even if you didn't reach your target weight the first time through—and I promise that you will eventually—I guarantee you'll notice at least one or two of those five dislikes about yourself start to either improve or disappear. Creating this short list will give you more reasons to celebrate at the end of 25Days—and the motivation to jump right back in and take on the next 25Days.

part two

....

THE 25DAYS DIET:
Your "Best You Blueprint"

chapter four

The Diet Rules You Need to Know

As my dad used to tell me, "Don't try to outthink your common sense."

When it comes to how and what you should eat on the 25Days program, it's exactly that: common sense. So if you just want to jump right into the program, I'm all for that. If you accept that what you'll be eating is balanced in such a way that it will convert your body from one that uses glycogen (carbohydrates stored in your muscles and liver) as its preferred source of energy into one that utilizes fat instead, then go for it. I admire that enthusiasm and wouldn't want to waste your time with any extra details. So, here's all you need to know:

The 25Days Diet *Simplified*!

For twenty-five days, you'll be alternating between two different daily meal plans: a **Primary Eating Day** on odd-numbered days and a **Secondary Eating Day** on even-numbered days.

+ On **Primary Days** (Days 1, 3, 5, 7, 9, and so on), you'll eat three meals and **two** snacks—one between each meal.

+ On **Secondary Days** (Days 2, 4, 6, 8, 10, and so on), you'll eat three meals and only **one** snack between lunch and dinner.

For Women

Every meal (breakfast, lunch, dinner) should ideally be a mix of:

+ 30 grams of lean protein

+ 20 grams of low-glycemic fibrous carbohydrates

+ 10 grams of healthy fats

+ 1 glass of water

Every snack should ideally be a mix of:

+ 15 grams of lean protein

+ 10 grams of low-glycemic fibrous carbohydrates

+ 5 grams of healthy fats

+ 1 glass of water

For Men

Every meal (breakfast, lunch, dinner) should ideally be a mix of:

+ 40 grams of lean protein

+ 30 grams of low-glycemic fibrous carbohydrates

+ 15 grams of healthy fats

+ 1 glass of water

Every snack should ideally be a mix of:

+ 20 grams of lean protein

+ 15 grams of low-glycemic fibrous carbohydrates

+ 7.5 grams of healthy fats

+ 1 glass of water

The Every-Five-Day Mind Meal Simplified

Every five days, you'll ignore these rules and eat what I call the **Every-Five-Day Mind Meal**—a meal that's nothing but low-glycemic starchy carbohydrates (a form of carbohydrate that doesn't raise your blood sugar level substantially but is still converted quickly into glucose).

+ For women, that meal should consist of no more than **80 grams** of low-glycemic starchy carbohydrates.

+ For men, that meal should consist of no more than **120 grams** of low-glycemic starchy carbohydrates.

+ For each meal or snack you eat properly on odd days (meaning, you've gotten in all of your nutrients and water), you'll give yourself 20 percent. Eat right for all three meals and two snacks, and you'll earn 100 percent.

+ For each meal or snack you eat properly on even days (meaning, you've gotten in all of your nutrients and water), you'll give yourself 25 percent. Eat right for all three meals and one snack, and you'll earn 100 percent.

That's it, but don't worry. In a perfect world, these are the exact numbers. This is the place I would love to see you at, but who lives in a perfect world? I know I don't.

You can't scream at the chef who prepared your chicken breast over vegetables for lunch that you can have only exactly 30 grams of protein. And it might not be possible or desirable for you to measure your food down to the last gram. The thing is, the entire purpose of 25Days is to provide you with a program that lives and breathes in the real world; one that allows you to eat healthy and be active without having to be so precise.

So you had rolls and butter at lunch with the boss, and you weren't supposed to—okay, so what? Quite honestly, if you continue to mess up to the point where you're slamming drinks at happy hour and having chili cheese fries, then, yes, you've just ruined the whole day. But in reality, if you botch a meal or snack once in a while, all it will cost you is 20 to 25 percent for the day—depending on how often you're allowed to eat that day.

If you stay the course, you may end up with a 75 percent grade for the day, but that's not a complete failure. It means only that you didn't hit every goal, but you can still be a success tomorrow. And if you score 100 percent with your workout, you'll still score higher than 85 percent for the day. You can be winning before the conversation is even over.

My point: if you're capable of following the program perfectly right down to the gram, then go for it. If you're prepared to measure out every bunch of broccoli and trim your chicken breast right down to the exact ounce, I'm not going to stop you. Otherwise just try to get as close to these numbers as you can. And don't worry: I'll show you how to take all of the thinking out of it in the next chapter.

That said, you can move on to the next chapter to learn about how to hit those ratios effortlessly every time—along with what you need to cut out of your diet. But if you're interested in a few details on why sticking to these rules is crucial for 25Days to work, then I'm ready to answer any questions you may have.

The 25Days Diet *Magnified*!

Q: *Why is each meal and snack divided up this way?*
A: The first reason behind the ratio of proteins, low-glycemic fibrous carbs, and healthy fats is to teach your body to utilize something that it's probably never done before. By eating in this way, you will quickly begin to train your body to prefer using fats for energy as opposed to carbohydrates. Once that switch has been flipped, your body will turn into a fat-burning machine all day long.

I also want you not just to be satisfied longer after each meal and snack, but equally important, I want your body to be in a greater state of healing from the workouts you'll be performing throughout the 25Days. By eating a high-protein, moderate-fat diet throughout the day, you'll be creating a healing metabolism for the cells that make up your muscles and other tissues, as well as a deeper sense of satiation.

Whenever I give lectures explaining this process, I like to take a whiteboard, put a tiny dot in the center, and then tell the audience that's what a carbohydrate molecule looks like. Then I draw a circle roughly the size of a basketball hoop and tell them that's what a protein molecule looks like. I want them to understand two things right off the bat:

1. The tiny ones are digested quickly, which causes your blood sugar level to rise. This triggers your pancreas to release insulin, which tells your cells to absorb any excess glucose in your bloodstream and store it as—you guessed it—unwanted fat.

2. The big ones are digested slowly, so they don't raise your insulin levels, which keeps that fat storage trigger from ever getting flipped.

That's why (even though the charts you'll find in the next chapter list the caloric values of the foods I'm suggesting you try) I'm not looking at any of your meals or snacks from a caloric standpoint. All I'm concerned about is how many grams of fat, protein, and carbohydrates (otherwise known as macronutrients) you're eating.

It's through maintaining this ratio of protein, low-glycemic carbs, and healthy fats that the 25Days Diet works. It's what will help give you more energy and ensure that your protein synthesis is higher and that you are kept in a constant state of healing. It's what will boost your lean muscle tissue and, as a result, increase your resting metabolic rate. It's what will keep your body in a perpetual anabolic state the entire twenty-five days, which is when your body's focused on building and preserving lean muscle tissue and burning fat as energy.

Q: Do I really need to be as strict with my snacks?
A: Yes. In my experience, I've found that some people put all their discipline into making sure they're eating the right amount of proteins, fibrous carbohydrates, and healthy fats in their meals but tend to skip that step when it comes to snacks.

Could you grab an apple in between meals and settle for that? You could, but I wouldn't. Not sticking with the right ratio makes it a lot easier to eat more than your body needs between meals. But more important, it's critical to keep your snacks as consistent as your meals so that your body continuously uses fat as energy. If you stray from that, it takes your body out of that fat-burning mode and makes it crave glycogen instead.

IF you find yourself not satiated or sluggish after having a snack . . .

THEN the chances are that you waited too long before eating it or your body is still identifying glycogen as its primary energy source.

What you're having is a blood sugar craving. That's normal—but I want you to recognize what's happening. Your body isn't looking for table sugar; it's looking for a source of reliable energy. By eating reliable sources of energy through protein, low-glycemic fibrous carbohydrates, and healthy fats, the energy your body needs is right there. But your brain is trying to retrain your body to prefer the options that you've presented it.

You're on the right track, and what you're feeling is a great indicator, so stay the course and press your way through. Do not—I repeat, do not—try to address the problem by reaching for more food.

Q: Does it matter when I eat?

A: It doesn't matter if you're an early eater or a late-to-the-plate kind of person. I don't mind what time you start eating, so long as you wait the appropriate amount of time between meals and snacks. Ideally, I'd like you to wait three hours after a meal to have your snack, and wait two hours after a snack to have your next meal. But if that sounds like a lot of computing, just have a meal or snack every three hours.

Q: *Do I have to drink water with every meal and snack?*

A: Absolutely. It's not about how having water will leave you feeling fuller. The real value is that every time you eat, your body immediately starts processing and assimilating what you've consumed—and it needs water to make that happen.

But don't think that anything poured into a glass counts. Having any liquid other than water with your meal is not only less helpful to your body but also detrimental because your body can't use other liquids as readily to help break down food.

Finally, if you're wondering how much water to have, I'm not going to be critical about how much you choose to drink. Most glasses range from 12 to 16 ounces, so if you don't feel like measuring every ounce, that's fine. Just make sure it's a decent-sized glass, and you should be just fine.

Q: *Why am I having one less snack every other day (on even-numbered days)?*

A: Because your body won't need as many calories on even-numbered days. The way the 25Days Workout is designed, you'll be doing a strength-training program on odd (or Primary) days and a cardio-conditioning program on even (or Secondary) days.

You might think that you would need more food on even days because you'll be doing a cardio-based workout. But the truth is: cardio is great, *but when you're done with cardio, cardio is done with you.* Your heart rate falls from an elevated state back to a resting state, and whatever calories you managed to burn in your workout are all you'll burn up to that point.

But on odd days, when you're strength training, your body processes energy differently. Afterward, your muscles need to repair themselves from your workout over the next day or so, which causes a spike in your resting metabolic rate. That metabolism boost causes you to burn more calories long after the hard work's done. On Secondary Days, you won't experience that same metabolism spike, so you'll need to pull out just a little bit of calories to compensate. That's why I recommend switching from two snacks down to one for the day.

Q: Okay, so what will really happen if I don't eat precisely as required?
A: Having more than what you're supposed to have, provided that you've done your workout for the day and you're eating healthy foods, isn't always a bad thing. 25Days isn't a calorie dance, but assuming you'll be honest about what type of foods you've eaten more of, then I'll be frank with you about this topic.

+ **If You Reached for More Protein, Healthy Fats, or Low-Glycemic Fibrous Carbs.** As long as you were hungry and you ate the right amount of the other two macronutrients, that's fine. If you do that, it doesn't change your grade, but you need to understand that you've eaten a certain amount of extra calories for the day. You need to be aware that if you feel like you're not reaching your goals fast enough, even though I'm not penalizing you for that meal or snack, you may be penalizing yourself in terms of possibly not seeing results as quickly.

+ **If You Reached for Sugar or Starchy Carbs.** On the other hand, if you were hungry, ate the right amount of proteins and fats, but you turned to the bad stuff (sugar or starchy carbs) instead of fibrous carbs, that's not fine. It's an automatic 20 percent deduction from your daily nutrition grade on a Primary Day and a 25 percent deduction on a Secondary Day.

    As a result, you'll have triggered your body to seek out glycogen for energy and hit your body with an insulin spike. It's impossible for your body to utilize fat when your insulin levels are elevated, so you'll have stopped the fat-burning machine we're trying to build. Also, any cravings you'll have managed to kick along the way—which can happen in as little as five days into the program—will return, so don't be shocked if you have to fight those cravings throughout the day and possibly into the next.

+ **If You Reached for Anything Other Than What I'm Asking You to Eat.** Meaning, if you did a complete replacement and the meal or snack you ate doesn't resemble at all what I've recommended, give yourself a *zero* for that meal or snack. I don't care if what you ate was the same calorically. If you substituted a meal or snack with a few cookies and a smoothie, you earn no points for that meal or snack.

Why? It's not just because you've taken yourself out of the fat-burning zone. By not eating any of the nutrients I'm advising you to have in each meal or snack—particularly large amounts of protein and healthy fat—you've also pulled your body out of a healing state. You just eliminated what it needs to recover from the program.

Q: *What if I eat healthy at every meal or snack, but I end up cheating in between?*

A: A lot of dieters love to do this because it's easier to justify throwing in an extra snack as a reward for eating healthy throughout the day. But the same issues I just discussed in the last question happen anytime you cheat: your body falls off the fat-burning wagon. If that's you, the program is not going to let you get away with that.

So here's how it works:

+ **If You Cheat on a Primary Day.** Eat anything bad for you beyond the allotted meals and snacks, and I want you to deduct 20 percent per serving for your entire nutrition grade at the end of the day.

+ **If You Cheat on a Secondary Day.** This is a worse penalty. If you decide to stray on a secondary day, deduct *25 percent* per serving off your entire nutrition grade.

What that boils down to is this: if you ate healthy at every meal or snack and earned 100 percent for the day but had three servings of cookies, you now have either a 40 percent grade for nutrition for the day (3 × 20 percent = –60 percent) or, even worse, a 25 percent grade for nutrition for the day (3 × 25 percent = –75 percent).

If you're still wanting to sneak in a little something from time to time, just take a look at the serving sizes of the types of foods you might consider when cheating. In a lot of cases, one serving might be just one cookie or a mere half cup of ice cream. When you measure it out (and if you're going to cheat, this is one time I'll expect you to be precise with measuring), the serving sizes of most bad-for-you foods aren't big. That's when you have to ask yourself if it's worth it to take an entire day's grade of 100 percent, earned by making all the right choices, and pull it down below 85 percent by having just one cookie.

Q: What if I eat an extra meal or snack but stay within the guidelines and eat the right amounts of protein, low-glycemic fibrous carbs, and healthy fats?

A: Believe it or not, I'm not going to give you a deduction, but I will give you a reminder.

First off, good on you for staying within the parameters of the kinds of foods you should be eating. Metabolically, your body will still be utilizing fat for energy and remaining in a state of healing. I can't penalize you because you've at least fed your body nutrients that it can use properly and kept your hormones in balance.

However, you need to understand that you've added additional calories to your system. If you begin to notice you're not seeing the numbers you were expecting on the scale, around your waistline, or with your dress size, just remember that it's most likely a result of that extra meal or snack you may be sneaking more often than you should.

Q: What if I decide to skip an entire meal or snack but still stay within the guidelines for the rest of my meals and snacks?

A: You earn absolutely nothing for that meal or snack. It's a complete meal deduction. Even if you ate healthy all day long, but you were supposed to eat three meals and two snacks, and you decided to skip one, you get credit only for four out of five meals—and you earn just 80 percent for the day.

The entire reason for eating the way I'm advising you to is to place your body in an anabolic, nitrogen-positive, high-protein synthesis state. You see, all three macronutrients (fats, proteins, and carbohydrates) contain carbon, hydrogen, and oxygen—but only protein contains nitrogen, which is required for muscle growth. When your body's nitrogen levels are positive (meaning, you're taking in more nitrogen than you're excreting), your body recovers and repairs itself faster. But when your body's nitrogen levels are negative, your body goes into a catabolic state, or starvation mode.

Eating on schedule keeps you in that anabolic state all day long. But when you skip a meal or snack, your body slides into a catabolic state. Then it stops burning fat and starts to feast on the lean muscle tissue we're trying to build—lean muscle that helps raise your metabolism so that you're always burning more calories at rest 24-7.

Q: What should I do if I'm eating healthy but didn't eat as much protein or fat as prescribed?
A: I'm fine with that—and I'll even let you take full credit for that meal or snack. But when you do that, you may feel hungrier either later on or in the middle of the night—especially if you've made that choice late in the day.

You may also experience an energy lull. From observations I've noticed with both myself and my clients over the years, there's about a three-to-six-hour period from the time you eat protein, depending on the type of protein you've consumed, to the time your body notices whether it's either had enough or needs more. That can cause some people to see a dip in their energy levels, so be aware that you may not have as much energy if you cut corners when it comes to protein.

The Every-Five-Day Mind Meal Magnified

Every fifth day, you're going to eat differently at your final meal. Instead of dividing your dinner to include protein, low-glycemic fibrous carbohydrates, and healthy fats, you're going to feast on a carb-rich dinner of nothing but low-glycemic, starchy carbohydrates (such as sweet potatoes, quinoa, oatmeal, brown rice, or quinoa pasta). You can use a minimal amount of healthy fats as a condiment, such as a drizzle of coconut oil or a little olive oil—but that's all.

- For women, the meal should contain no more than **80 grams** of low-glycemic starchy carbohydrates.

- For men, the meal should contain no more than **120 grams** of low-glycemic starchy carbohydrates.

If you're worried about the calories you're consuming, don't be. Calorically, you'll be eating the same amount found in one of the program's typical dinners. The reason I stress that is because I don't want guilt to make you think this is a meal you can skip. You won't be getting any extra results by doing so. In fact, your results will only grind to a stop.

Why a Mind Meal? As you move through 25Days, it's important to recalibrate both your body and your brain by placing them in a state of hyperhealing. Eating low-glycemic starchy carbohydrates (something your body hasn't had for five days) does exactly that—in more ways than you can imagine.

The first thing you'll be doing by eating a Mind Meal is resetting two hunger hormones: leptin and ghrelin. Leptin is responsible for suppressing your appetite by telling the brain it has enough energy available, while ghrelin increases your appetite by signaling hunger to the brain. The Mind Meal works like this: after five days, your body starts noticing a caloric deficit, which causes your leptin level to drop and your ghrelin level to rise.

It's a hormone imbalance that not only makes you hungrier but also causes your metabolism to slow down to conserve stored energy. Throwing in a Mind Meal every five days provides you with just enough food to reset your hormone levels. Your brain immediately believes that everything's fine, which keeps your metabolism raised and your body utilizing fat for energy.

Your Mind Meal also plays a key role in lowering cortisol (the stress hormone guilty of using your lean muscle tissue for energy) and replenishing serotonin (the feel-good hormone that improves your mood).

After five days, there will be a slight increase in your cortisol levels and a decrease in serotonin, due to your eating fewer carbohydrates. Having a Mind Meal containing nothing but carbohydrates shuts down the release of cortisol while normalizing your serotonin level to a place that will help you curb any carb cravings you may have over the next few days.

Just as important, the Mind Meal restores your glycogen level using low-glycemic starchy carbohydrates that are easier on your pancreas. These types of carbohydrates pull in a lot of water as they significantly increase the glycogen level within your muscles. That causes your body to slip into a state of hyperhealing, one that speeds up the process of repairing broken-down muscle fibers. And while you're asleep, it increases the release of insulin-like growth factor 1 (IGF-1), a protein that exerts a powerful anabolic effect on the body and aids in weight loss. That hyperhealing is why most people wake up the next day feeling significantly more energetic and ready to go.

But don't expect that energy boost while you're eating it. Your Mind Meal may give you that Thanksgiving Day feeling. Will it make you tired? Probably. But it will be a very soothing feeling caused by the increased serotonin and dopamine in your system. I've even had some clients notice how they can feel their temperature rise from their body's hormonal response. So just enjoy the ride and know that you're not just satisfying your appetite—you're also resetting your brain and body to take on the next five-day block.

Q: What happens if I skip a Mind Meal?
A: As I mentioned earlier in this chapter, missing any meal or snack earns you 0 percent because you'll be switching your body from a fat-burning anabolic state to a muscle-burning catabolic state. But missing this Mind Meal comes with another major disadvantage: it can cause you to skid into a plateau. After five days, your body will be exhausted from a hard five-day block, and you need to eat it. It's either rest—or regret.

Q: Hey! Why do guys get to eat 50 percent more in this meal than women—compared with eating only 25 percent or so more than women during the other meals and snacks in the program?

A: The answer is simple: it comes down to muscle. If you're a woman, I don't want you to feel cheated, but the truth is that men build muscle tissue faster and typically have more muscle on their frame. That being said, all of that muscle acts like a sponge to absorb more glycogen at a much faster rate.

With less muscle, women have less of a sponge to rely on, so they don't store as much glycogen—and it doesn't happen as quickly. Because of this, women tend to typically see more of the negative effects of eating a lot of carbs the day after. If you eat more than what I've recommended, any excess is going to show up as bloating, which, even though it's a natural and temporary effect, could turn off some women from sticking with the program long enough to create a new neurological pattern.

Q: What about counting fiber? Isn't that essential for living a healthy lifestyle?

A: It absolutely is. The benefits of fiber are numerous, from assisting with weight loss and promoting digestive health to controlling blood sugar levels to prevent type 2 diabetes and lowering cholesterol by as much as 10 to 15 percent, which can reduce your risk of heart disease and stroke.

One of the many amazing side benefits of 25Days is that you're eating nonstarchy, fibrous carbohydrates in every meal and snack. Because of that, the odds are that you'll most likely meet or exceed your fiber requirements for the day without having to even think about it.

chapter five

The Diet Put-Ins/the Cut-Outs

N ow that you know the numbers needed in each meal and snack—
the ratio that will turn your body into a fat-burning machine
night and day—it's time to show you how to hit those numbers
without having to think too hard.

But I don't want you to get too hung up on serving sizes. Whether a
person eats five ounces of fish instead of four ounces isn't the issue for
most people—and it's definitely not the reason they may be overweight
or not reaching their health and fitness goals.

Instead, I just want you to get close. I just want you to eyeball what
you're eating as best you can. Your first 25Days is about getting used to
the parameters of the program, and at some point, you can get picky
about serving sizes. But for now . . .

The 25Days Diet Put-Ins/Cut-Outs *Simplified*!

For convenience, use the charts in this chapter as a way to quickly pick
servings of protein, low-glycemic fibrous carbs, and healthy fats. Even
though you're free to eat what you wish, try to pick foods that are higher
up on the lists. The higher you choose on each list, the more nutritional
value your brain and body will receive. There are five types of foods that I
want you to avoid for twenty-five days. I call them "neural no-no's." They
are, in no particular order:

+ Soda (that includes diet sodas, "zero" sodas, and even soda water)

- Sweets and sugar

- Processed foods

- Alcohol

- Fried food of any kind

You are allowed to eat the following free-for-all foods without restriction:

- Any green vegetable (broccoli, bell peppers, cucumbers, asparagus, cabbage, snow peas, and so on)

- Any leafy greens (such as spinach, kale, arugula, lettuce)

- Cauliflower

- Strawberries

- Peaches

- Grapefruit

- Apples

- Cherries

Simple, right? If you're ready to start, just turn to page 56 in this chapter and use the charts provided to put together any variety of meals and snacks. However, if you stick around a little longer, I'll explain why certain foods aren't allowed on the 25Days Diet and why others can be eaten all day long guilt free.

The 25Days Diet Put-Ins/Cut-Outs *Magnified*!

The thing I need you to think about when it comes to your nutrition is that this diet works in concert with the exercise program I've created. I want you to build your meals and snacks in the exact order given:

The Put-Ins

1. FOCUS ON PROTEIN FIRST

I want you to always pick your protein source first. This is the nutrient that deserves the most attention, meaning, I don't want you to go into any meal or snack wondering where your carbs are. That protein source should set the tone for everything else on your plate.

The thing to understand is that there's a difference between a hunger craving and a blood sugar craving. A hunger craving is a sensation of actually needing food, while a blood sugar craving occurs when your blood sugar level drops. By having greater amounts of protein in every meal and snack, you'll reduce your hunger cravings, so you can check that off your list of concerns while on 25Days.

Protein is also the one macronutrient among the three that your body can't store as protein or the amino acids it contains (the compounds that are the building blocks of protein and critical for both tissue repair and maintaining your muscles). That's why it's crucial that protein is present at every eating opportunity to ensure that your body always has what it needs to heal.

2. FILL IN YOUR FATS

The next thing to focus on are your fats. Because you'll be balancing out the rest of your plate with primarily low-glycemic fibrous carbs, your body will experience a relatively low glycemic response from the carbohydrates that you're eating. Not only is this easier on your pancreas, but it tells your body to begin seeking out and breaking down fat as an energy source instead of glycogen and carbohydrates.

By adding enough healthy fats into each meal and snack, your brain will begin to use—and prefer—those fats as a healthy energy source, so you'll receive a constant, even feeling of mental awareness and sustained energy throughout the day. That means the typical energy highs and lows you're used to experiencing during the day when eating carbs will disappear.

3. FINISH WITH LOW-GLYCEMIC FIBROUS CARBS

Finally, add your carbs, but make sure they're the right ones. Why a lot of people fail on typical diet and exercise programs is that when you start talking about carbohydrates, people immediately think about their favorites, such as bread, pasta, potatoes, and rice.

The carb ratios I'm asking you to stick with during each meal and snack may seem low. But for 25Days to work, and what determines how well you succeed on it, depends on the foods you're choosing to fulfill those carbohydrate requirements each day—they must come from low-glycemic fibrous carbohydrates.

You see, every carbohydrate-based food has an effect on how high it elevates your blood sugar levels after you eat it. That effect is known as the glycemic index (GI). Every food you eat falls between 0 and 100. The higher the number, the higher it elevates your blood sugar levels.

Protein-based foods such as eggs, meats, and fish don't even rank on the GI scale, but carbs are a different story. Foods low on the GI scale (such as most fruits and vegetables, legumes such as beans and lentils, most dairy products, whole grains, and nuts) barely raise your blood sugar level at all because they release glucose slowly and steadily. Foods high on the GI scale (such as white bread, most white rices, and most breakfast cereals) elevate your sugar level out of control because they release glucose rapidly.

Having you stick with low-glycemic fibrous carbs will not only keep you feeling fuller longer thanks to all the extra fiber they provide, but also they take a lot longer to digest. That slow and steady release of glucose keeps your blood sugar level even and prevents your body from releasing insulin as often, so you're never storing excess calories in places you don't want them to show.

In addition, fibrous carbs are abundant in vitamins, minerals, phytochemicals, and other nutrients, as well as fiber. That bonus means most of the carbs you'll be eating will pass through your intestines instead of being absorbed, keeping your digestive system healthy while keeping you from storing any unwanted calories.

The Cut-Outs

Are there a few foods you're not allowed on the 25Days Diet? Absolutely. But these obvious choices aren't strictly off limits because of their extra calories and how they negatively impact your overall health. They're officially what I like to call the five Neural No-No's because of how they also interfere with how quickly and easily you can rewire your brain and shift it toward a healthier lifestyle.

The Five Neural No-No's

1. NO SODA

That includes no "diet sodas," "zero" sodas, and even soda water.

The thing I always ask my clients if they're having a hard time cutting back on soda is have them tell me how much of their body is made up of carbonated water. Here's a hint: zero. Your body isn't made up of carbonated water—it's made up of H_2O.

Beyond the obvious extra calories in many sodas, I have clients stay away from diet sodas and even club soda, plain seltzer, and tonic water with good reason. Because of the gas formed by carbonation, any carbonated beverage you choose isn't absorbed as readily, so it's never the best choice for staying hydrated. To make matters worse, even if you are stepping away from sugary drinks because of their calories, most likely you're substituting them with a no-calorie or low-calorie soda that uses other chemicals to achieve that sweet taste you're craving.

Why It's a Neural No-No. The artificial sweeteners—particularly aspartame, saccharin, and sucralose—found in many diet sodas and drinks have been shown to alarm your brain of an impending caloric crisis, which may increase your impulsivity. Researchers at the University of South Dakota[*] found that drinking soda containing artificial sweeteners increased the likelihood that subjects would choose a smaller short-term

---

[*]X. T. Wang and Robert D. Dvorak, "Sweet Future: Fluctuating Blood Glucose Levels Affect Future Discounting," *Psychological Science* 21, no. 2 (2010): 183–88, doi:10.1177/0956797609358096, Epub January 20, 2010.

reward rather than a larger reward in the future, suggesting that artificial sweeteners affect your brain's ability to make decisions.

IF *you desire soda every so often . . .*

THEN *increase how much water you're drinking per meal and snack. When properly hydrated, most soda drinkers tend to lose their desire for soda. What I also try to get clients to do is switch over to lemon water.*

But if drinking more water or having lemon water doesn't cut it, opt for some form of sugar-free, all-natural fizzy water. And by *all natural*, I mean nothing with aspartame or anything artificial—it must be sweetened with either stevia, a natural sweetener made from the stevia plant, or monk fruit extract, a low-glycemic natural sweetener made from monk fruit, an Asian gourd—both are easily found in any health-food aisle. What people don't realize is that a lot of artificial sweeteners still raise insulin levels, which will prevent your body from utilizing fat as energy. Personally, I'm not a fan of these types of alternative waters, but if I can't stop you, then do it the way that is least damaging to you.

If none of these suggestions does the trick and you insist on having a glass of soda now and then, here's the deal: for every serving you drink, it's an automatic 20 percent deduction from your daily nutrition grade on a Primary Day and 25 percent from your daily nutrition grade on a Secondary Day.

I also need you to understand that a carbonated drink is going to cause bloating, either from the gas or the sodium present in most unflavored carbonated water. Plus, know that you won't be able to get as lean as you would like.

2. NO SUGAR AND SWEETS

That means anything made with table sugar, syrup, molasses, and even honey is not allowed. That goes for every sweetener out there, which all cause a glycemic response that elevates blood sugar. The only sweeteners you're allowed to have on 25Days are stevia or monk fruit.

Ready for some honesty? I have a sweet tooth. And at any given moment, there's nothing more I would rather do than head to the bakery down the street from me and get a dozen homemade salted chocolate chip cookies. And because I've already reached my goals and use the 25Days program to maintain my health and fitness, I have a few (not twelve!) cookies once in a while at the right time during the 25Days journey—and you will too. But for now, I don't want you to do that because it would be a deterrent from where you want to go.

It comes down to this: *anything that raises your insulin level is going to negate your body's ability to utilize fat as energy—period.*

That's exactly what sugar, sweets, and any form of simple carbohydrate do. Because these foods are broken down and absorbed into your bloodstream quickly, they cause your blood sugar level to spike.

Anything that ranks high on the glycemic index—the ranking system from 0 to 100 that measures how quickly or slowly a carbohydrate-containing food increases your blood glucose level—can cause your insulin to spike. But for now, eliminating the most obvious choices directly at their source is what I want you to do.

Another reason sugar and sweets are off the list is that whenever you increase insulin, it triggers a release of serotonin, which can leave you feeling more sluggish and tired afterward. Mostly, it keeps you from reaching your goal of losing unwanted body fat in two ways: it causes you to store more fat, and it deprives you of the energy you need not just to accomplish your workouts but also to feel good throughout the day.

Why They're a Neural No-No. The main reason is that you'll find it much harder to forge a healthier neurological pattern, because eating these types of foods floods your system with dopamine, which is what we're trying to regulate and get under control. Eat too much—or even just a little—of them, and you'll receive less of a dopamine response at the end of the day, when you want it most.

Eating large amounts of fructose, which includes cane sugar (or sucrose) and high-fructose corn syrup, has also been shown to alter your brain's ability to learn and retain information. Researchers at the University of California, Los Angeles (UCLA),* discovered that a diet steadily high in fructose slows the brain, hampering memory and learning, in as little as six weeks.

IF you have a difficult time cutting out sweets . . .
THEN look at your hydration and healthy fats.

How bad your sugar cravings may be will depend on where you are along the 25Days journey. During your first few days, when you're getting sugar out of your system, I won't lie: it can be a challenge. Especially if you are a big sweets person. If that's you, then no amount of healthy fats is going to cure that feeling.

Understanding what's going on is the best place to start. When your body craves sugar, it's searching for energy and failing to recognize fats as the preferred source of energy. By doing the right thing and adding healthy fats, you'll be giving it the energy it's looking for, but from a much healthier source.

That said, try raising the amount of healthy fats in each meal by adding a slice of avocado or something else that provides a few extra grams of healthy fats. Mind you, this isn't any hard-and-fast number, since everyone responds differently when incorporating healthy fats into his or her system, but it's one I've found works with both me and my clients.

Also, cravings and dehydration go hand in hand. So if you're craving sweets, take an honest look at your hydration for the day. If you've been drinking the minimum requirement I've asked of you, which is one glass per meal and snack, I want you to increase that. Being overly hydrated helps to curb the body's cravings as well.

---

*Elaine Schmidt, "This Is Your Brain on Sugar: UCLA Study Shows High-Fructose Diet Sabotages Learning, Memory," news release, May 15, 2012, http://newsroom.ucla.edu/releases/this-is-your-brain-on-sugar-ucla-233992; Rahul Agrawal and Fernando Gomez-Pinilla, "'Metabolic Syndrome' in the Brain: Deficiency in Omega-3 Fatty Acid Exacerbates Dysfunctions in Insulin Receptor Signalling and Cognition," *Journal of Physiology* 590, no. 10 (2012): 2485–99.

But in those rare moments when you absolutely, positively have to eat something sweet, then I have two things I need you to do:

One: for every serving you eat, it's an automatic 20 percent deduction from your daily nutrition grade on a Primary Day and 25 percent from your daily nutrition grade on a Secondary Day.

Two: I want your craving to do the least amount of damage possible. So if you have to eat a serving of something sweet, then have it on an odd-numbered day and consume it immediately following your Primary Day workout. Elevating your insulin levels at the very end of a high-intensity workout will help your muscles repair and recover, since a rise in insulin increases protein synthesis.

Finally, just remember: surrendering to your sweet tooth will undoubtedly prevent you from getting as lean as you want, so give 25Days enough time to curb those cravings.

3. NO PROCESSED FOODS

If you can't grow it, fish it out of an ocean or lake, or raise it on a farm, it's not allowed for 25Days.

With 25Days, I want you eating foods of which you know, beyond a shadow of a doubt, what to expect—something that's nearly impossible to do when you incorporate processed foods into your diet.

See, processed foods tend to be sneaky, because each has its own collection of artificial ingredients. Unless you're a kung fu master at interpreting a product's ingredient's list, odds are you may not have any idea what you're eating. And despite what it might say on the package (since a lot of processed foods love to tout being healthier choices), many raise your blood sugar levels and trigger the release of insulin, which is why they're among the five Neural No-No's.

Why They're a Neural No-No. Believe it or not, it turns out that TV dinners could be as addictive to your brain as drugs are. In a recent study,* researchers looked at the pharmacokinetic properties of highly processed foods. What they discovered is that the refined carbohydrates in highly processed foods have the same characteristics as addictive drugs, in that both are rapidly absorbed in high doses by the body. This response could be the reason why more people are likely to have addictive-like eating when it comes to highly processed foods.

IF you need to have something processed . . .

THEN ask yourself why you're reaching for it in the first place.

Often, the entire reason you're grabbing that frozen meal or snack bar is that it's convenient. But the truth of the matter is, the 25Days Diet couldn't be any more convenient.

As you'll come to discover later in this chapter, all the charts I've designed will make it effortless for you to plan your meals and snacks. That's also why, for chapter 6, I collaborated with one of the top healthy chefs in the country to create easy recipes that will accommodate the busiest individual out there. You can stick them in your fridge or freeze them in portion sizes.

However, if you find yourself reaching for a processed food item because you have no time, it's an automatic 20 percent deduction per serving from your daily nutrition grade on a Primary Day and 25 percent on a Secondary Day.

4. NO ALCOHOL

I won't get into the many reasons already known why too much alcohol is bad for your health. Instead, I'll just explain why it negates what you're trying to do on the 25Days program.

---

*Erica M. Schulte, Nicole M. Avena, and Ashley N. Gearhardt, "Which Foods May Be Addictive? The Roles of Processing, Fat Content, and Glycemic Load," *PLoS One*, February 18, 2015, doi:10.1371/journal.pone.0117959.

The thing to realize about alcohol is that it that raises your blood sugar and stops your body from utilizing fat as energy. It also creates a surplus of calories that your body can't use in any way, so it stores them as unwanted body fat.

But what alcohol also does is toxify your liver, your body's filter system responsible for processing, assimilating, and storing most of your nutrients. Alcohol inhibits the organ, so that it processes things at a much slower rate. That means all of the good things you're trying to give your body through the food you're eating become much harder to absorb.

Why It's a Neural No-No. Dopamine is the key to making the 25Days program work. But a new study has recently revealed how alcohol may also interfere with the brain's ability to use the neurotransmitter. When researchers in Germany* examined the brains of deceased alcoholics, they discovered fewer D1 dopamine receptors, sites in the brain where dopamine binds and stimulates the brain cells (neurons) responsible for delivering nerve impulses. With fewer receptors, the brain becomes less responsive to dopamine, as well as less efficient at both producing and transporting dopamine.

> **IF** you feel obligated to have "one" drink . . .
>
> **THEN** ask yourself why you feel that way.
>
> ———————
>
> I've been in every possible business and entertainment situation you can imagine. I'm constantly around agents and producers, spending time at wrap parties for major movie premieres and concert tours, where drinking is prevalent. But I've never been in a position where I felt I had to have a drink or where anybody had a problem with my not having one.
>
> The truth is, if you "have" to have a drink, then we're

---

*N. Hirth et al., "Convergent Evidence from Alcohol-Dependent Humans and Rats for a Hyperdopaminergic State in Protracted Abstinence," *Proceedings of the National Academy of Sciences of the United States of America* 113, no. 11 (2016): 3024–29, doi:10.1073/pnas.1506012113, Epub February 22, 2016.

talking about something else here. But if that's not you, and addiction is off the table, and this is simply a peer pressure issue, that's another matter. The reality is, it's your choice, and you don't have to have a drink.

That being said, there are ways around it. The one option I tell a lot of my clients to do is to order your own drink at the bar, ask the bartender to put some water in a highball glass with a lemon slice, olives, or whatever you need to dress it up to make it look like you're having a vodka tonic, and that's it. It's going to help you stick with your program.

But if that isn't an option, my one go-to is a single glass of red wine. Red wine is high in resveratrol, an antioxidant that has been shown to improve cardiovascular health by lowering bad cholesterol (low-density lipoprotein, or LDL). It's also been proven to help keep blood vessels open and free of plaque and could boost your brain function by preventing the formation of beta-amyloid protein, the main ingredient in the plaque found in the brains of patients with Alzheimer's disease.

Although it's the least of all evils, alcohol is still a sugar. It packs 7 calories per gram of something your body can't use. In addition, alcohol is also a depressant. Because the entire 25Days program is spun around healthy brain function, alcohol is one of the worst neural no-no's to cheat with, and I consider it much worse than having a cookie. That's why for every alcoholic drink you have, it's an automatic 20 percent deduction from your daily nutrition grade on a Primary Day and 25 percent on a Secondary Day.

5. NO FRIED FOODS OF ANY KIND

In addition to clogging arteries and increasing your overall risk of developing type 2 diabetes,[*] chronically elevated blood pressure, or hyperten-

*Leah E. Cahill et al., "Fried-Food Consumption and Risk of Type 2 Diabetes and Coronary Artery Disease: A Prospective Study in 2 Cohorts of US Women and Men," *American Journal of Clinical Nutrition* 100, no. 2 (2014): 667–75, doi:10.3945/ajcn.114.084129, Epub June 18, 2014.

sion,* and even Alzheimer's, fried foods also deprive cells of oxygen, which accelerates the aging process and has been linked to many forms of cancer.

But what concerns me most about fried foods is what they do to your heart. According to research,† men who ate fried foods one to three times weekly had an 18 percent increased risk of developing heart failure. Bump those numbers to four to six times a week, and that number rises to 25 percent. Eat fried foods every day, and your risk of heart failure is a whopping 68 percent.

Why They're a Neural No-No. Even though eating plenty of healthy fats keep your brain healthy, it turns out that consuming saturated fats in the form of fried foods can make it difficult for your brain to control what you eat. A new study‡ from the Second University of Naples in Naples, Italy, found that meals high in saturated fat—particularly fried foods—cause inflammation in the brain and affect the hypothalamus, the part of the brain that regulates hunger.

***IF** you crave fried foods . . .*

***THEN** remember what you're really craving.*

———————

When it comes to anything of the fried variety, the irony is that it's typically not the food itself that's the problem. You're not dying for the taste of a ring-shaped onion, that piece of chicken, or a slice of French-fried potato—you're craving the crap that's either wrapped around it or cooked inside it.

Most fried stuff is high in saturated fat, but to make mat-

---

*C. Sayon-Orea et al., "ReportedFriedFoodConsumption and the Incidence of Hypertension in a Mediterranean Cohort: The SUN (Seguimiento Universidad de Navarra) Project," *British Journal of Nutrition* 112, no. 6 (September 28, 2014): 984–91, doi:10.1017/S0007114514001755.

†Cahill et al., "Fried-Food Consumption and Risk of Type 2 Diabetes and Coronary Artery Disease: A Prospective Study in 2 Cohorts of US Women and Men." *American Journal of Clinical Nutrition* 100, no. 2 (2014): 667–75, doi:10.3945/ajcn.114.084129, Epub June 18, 2014.

‡Emanuela Viggiano et al., "Effects of an High-Fat Diet Enriched in Lard or in Fish Oil on the Hypothalamic Amp-Activated Protein Kinase and Inflammatory Mediators,"*Frontiers in Cellular Neuroscience* 10 (June 9, 2016): 150, doi:10.3389/fncel.2016.00150.

ters worse, it's almost always covered in breading. It's the breading—not the food itself—that you're addicted to in the first place. If you don't believe me, take any food you typically enjoy fried and fry it up plain—without breading.

I know you'll tell me it doesn't taste the same, and you'd be right. But it's not just because you've removed something delicious that makes it less tasty. It's because it doesn't give you a spike in your blood sugar. You're addicted to the carbohydrates wrapped around those foods, the same ones that trigger a higher insulin response, which in turn causes you to store more body fat.

To make matters worse, the white flour used in most fried foods can also intoxicate your liver in the same way that alcohol does, preventing it from properly doing its job of processing and delivering nutrients throughout your body. That's why for every serving you eat, it's an automatic 20 percent deduction from your daily nutrition grade on a Primary Day and 25 percent on a Secondary Day.

The Free-for-All List

Americans aren't overweight because people are eating too many peaches. And when was the last time you saw anyone on a talk show crying herself a river about how fat she got putting away too much spinach? Exactly! That's why when it comes to the following low-glycemic fruits and vegetables, you'll have the freedom to eat as much as you feel your body needs:

+ Any green vegetable (broccoli, bell peppers, cucumbers, asparagus, cabbage, snow peas, etc.)

+ Any leafy greens (spinach, kale, arugula, lettuce, etc.)

+ Cauliflower

+ Strawberries

+ Peaches

- Grapefruit

- Apples

- Cherries

These are the foods I'm allowing you to eat without restriction for several reasons. The first is that all of them are low-glycemic, fibrous foods that are ideal for keeping you satiated during the day. The second reason? None of them triggers the release of dopamine to any great extent, so it never will affect your daily dopamine levels in a way that waters down that aha! moment I want you to experience at the end of the day when you receive your grade.

That's why I never want you worrying about weighing your broccoli, asparagus, cabbage—whatever it is. That's why I'll never tell you that you can have only so much cucumber in your salad. Have as much as you like. You can eat it by the bucketload because it won't be a problem.

These are also great foods to use when you're more susceptible to mindless snacking. Instead of putting tempting foods in front of you when watching a movie (or any activity where you often find yourself typically reaching for food), most of the free-for-all foods fit that crunchy profile, so they'll feel satisfying from an oral fixation standpoint.

I only have two things about the free-for-all list that I want you to understand:

- **Don't Eat These Foods in Place of Your Meals and Snacks.** You can have any of these foods *in addition to* your meals and snacks—and you can have as much of them as you want.

- **Work These Foods into Your Meal Preparation.** Try to figure out ways to garnish your meals and snacks with these free-for-all foods at every turn. Not only will you be adding extra flavor to what you're eating, but you'll be adding volume to them as well—all without changing anything that would stop your body from continuing to utilize fat for energy.

The 25Days Food Charts

Welcome to something different. Something I can promise will not only make it easy for you to create a wide variety of 25Days meals and snacks but also will unexpectedly have you making even better choices regarding what you eat from this point forward. That's because the charts in 25Days do more than just deliver information—they are meant to teach you, which is something that most charts never bother to do.

They Remove the Math

What makes my charts different—and defies others you've probably relied upon in the past—is that mine do most of the math for you. After all, I figured it's the least I can do, since I'm asking you to be specific regarding how many grams of protein, healthy fats, and low-glycemic fibrous carbs are in your meals and snacks.

So instead of listing foods in the "typical" average serving sizes the way nearly all lifestyle and diet books do—you know: all meats listed in 3-ounce portions, and every vegetable listed in 1-cup serving sizes—I've recalculated each portion size so that the number of grams per serving is as close to 5 grams, 10 grams, or the exact number of grams you need to eat of a nutrient in that meal or snack.

Here's how it works: let's say you're female, and it's dinnertime, which means you need to eat 30 grams of protein, 20 grams of low-glycemic fibrous carbs, and 10 grams of healthy fats. Here's all you have to do:

- ✦ **Pick a Protein from the Chart.** I've approximated the exact amount you would need to eat to get 30 grams for women or 40 grams for men.

- ✦ **Pick a Healthy Fat from the Chart.** I've adjusted the serving sizes in 5-gram portions, so you can add two servings to reach your 10-gram goal.

- ✦ **Pick a Low-Glycemic Fibrous Carb from the Chart.** I've adjusted the serving sizes in 5-gram or 10-gram portions, so you can throw in two to four helpings to reach your 20-gram goal.

What about snacks? Because the protein, fats, and carbs required for snacks are exactly *half* of what you're expected to put into your meals, it's just as easy to cut your protein portion sizes in half to know what to eat in between meals.

They Make It Easier to Choose

I prefer to have my clients see their food choices ranging from best to good as opposed to being listed alphabetically. (I won't say best to *worst*, because anything on the charts is still a smart choice.) As you use the charts to decide what to eat, I suggest that you choose as high up on each list as possible.

But know this: if you choose anything from the middle, or even at the bottom, that's fine too. What I want you to be aware of is what you're getting from your foods. Food sources that are lower on the list are down there for different reasons, whether it's because they contain less fiber, trigger a greater insulin release, have less nutritional value, or are higher in saturated fats.

Mind you, it's not an exact science—but I find it works.

If not having things arranged in alphabetical order makes things more difficult for you, I get it. But that's sort of the point. I want you to start thinking about your foods in the way you should be thinking about them: what they're providing your body nutrient-wise. I want you to start getting used to going for the foods that give your mind and body greater nutritional value.

So it might be a little confusing at first, and I'll admit that I expect you to be sometimes a little annoyed when you're searching like crazy for a particular food. But as you find each food, you'll get a better sense of how it fares versus other foods you could be choosing instead. It will open your eyes to where your foods truly rank.

They're in the Right Order

I've also placed the charts in the order you'll need them, starting with:

+ **Group 1:** proteins (always the first thing to consider when creating or evaluating your meals)

+ **Group 2:** healthy fats (for healthy brain function and to get you lean!)

+ **Group 3:** low-glycemic fibrous carbs (the number one choice for carbs)

+ **Group 4:** fruits (best limited to snacks alone)

+ **Group 5:** dairy (though viable options as a protein source, for optimal weight loss, should be kept at a minimum)

+ **Group 6:** starchy carbs (to be used only for your Every-Five-Day Mind Meal)

Each of the charts is arranged so that the macronutrient you need to focus on is right there front and center. But if you look to the right, you're also going to notice how many grams of the other two macronutrients are in that food as well. For example, you'll notice that many protein choices also have a certain amount of fat. Or that certain carbohydrates and fats also have a little bit of protein.

I don't want you to concern yourself with these numbers or add them into the equation in any way. They're not enough to mess up your diet or the 25Days program. But I've listed them so you will understand that they're in there and they do contribute to the overall caloric balance of each food.

GROUP 1: LEAN PROTEIN

The more valuable the protein you take in, the more useful it is in creating protein synthesis and boosting the healing process. That's why when I work with my clients, I try to get them to look at the usable value of the protein they take in.

See, although a single gram of protein always contains 4 calories, the amount of protein that your body can digest and use for healing and building lean muscle isn't always 100 percent. That's why I've arranged the protein choices by their biological values (BV), a measurement used to determine what percentage of a given nutrient (in this case, protein) is *actually* utilized by the body.

Eggs rank number one because 100 percent of the protein within them gets assimilated and used by your body—not a gram goes to waste. Every other source—fish, chicken, beef, pork, and so forth—is rated according to how digestible it is compared with egg protein. But don't worry, even the lowest choices on the chart have a BV of 80 percent, meaning, your body uses 80 percent of what you've eaten and the rest goes to waste. That said, whenever possible, pick from highest to lowest.

Just for the ladies: these portion sizes are at the *highest* end of the scale. Even though you're allowed up to 30 grams of protein in each meal and up to 15 grams in each snack, listen to your body.

Protein is the most long-term satiating of all macronutrients, so if you're finding yourself hungry (truly hungry—not having a sugar craving), then it makes sense to eat the maximum grams of protein. However, if you feel satisfied and full, by all means box up the rest for leftovers.

LEAN PROTEIN

WOMEN: 30g. each meal/15g. each snack
MEN: 40g. each meal/20g. each snack

	Serving Size	Protein (g.)	Calories	Total Fat (g.)	Saturated Fat (g.)	Carbs (g.)
Egg (whole)	1 large	6	70	5	2	0
Egg (white)	1 large	4	17	0	0	0
Sashimi (yellowfin tuna)	F: 4 oz. (4 pieces) M: 6 oz. (6 pieces)	F: 28 M: 42	F: 121 M: 182	F: 1 M: 2	F: 0 M: 0	F: 0 M: 0
Sashimi (yellowtail)	F: 4 oz. (4 pieces) M: 6 oz. (6 pieces)	F: 29 M: 43	F: 167 M: 251	F: 6 M: 9	F: 1 M: 2	F: 0 M: 0
Tuna (bluefin, baked)	F: 4 oz. M: 6 oz.	F: 26 M: 40	F: 163 M: 245	F: 6 M: 8	F: 1 M: 2	F: 0 M: 0
Sashimi (salmon)	F: 5 oz. (5 pieces) M: 7 oz. (7 pieces)	F: 30 M: 42	F: 200 M: 287	F: 8 M: 12	F: 1.5 M: 2.5	F: 0 M: 0
Atlantic salmon, baked	F: 4 oz. M: 6 oz.	F: 29 M: 43	F: 206 M: 309	F: 9 M: 14	F: 1 M: 2	F: 0 M: 0
Trout, baked	F: 4 oz. M: 6 oz.	F: 30 M: 45	F: 216 M: 324	F: 10 M: 15	F: 2 M: 3	F: 0 M: 0
Striped bass, baked	F: 4.5 oz. M: 6 oz.	F: 29 M: 39	F: 158 M: 211	F: 4 M: 5	F: 1 M: 1	F: 0 M: 0
Halibut, baked	F: 5 oz. M: 7 oz.	F: 29 M: 40	F: 155 M: 217	F: 3 M: 5	F: 1 M: 1	F: 0 M: 0
Sea bass, baked	F: 4 oz. M: 6 oz.	F: 27 M: 40	F: 140 M: 211	F: 3 M: 4	F: 1 M: 1	F: 0 M: 0
Flounder, baked	F: 4.5 oz. M: 6 oz.	F: 31 M: 41	F: 150 M: 200	F: 2 M: 3	F: 0 M: 0.5	F: 0 M: 0
Sole, baked	F: 4.5 oz. M: 6 oz.	F: 31 M: 41	F: 150 M: 200	F: 2 M: 3	F: 0 M: 1	F: 0 M: 0
Scallops, steamed or broiled	5 scallops	10	70	2	0	2

	Serving Size	Protein (g.)	Calories	Total Fat (g.)	Saturated Fat (g.)	Carbs (g.)
Shrimp	F: 4.5 oz. M: 6 oz.	F: 29 M: 39	F: 152 M: 202	F: 2 M: 3	F: 0.5 M: 1	F: 2 M: 3
Catfish, baked	F: 6 oz. M: 8 oz.	F: 31 M: 42	F: 178 M: 238	F: 5 M: 7	F: 1 M: 2	F: 0 M: 0
Haddock, baked	F: 4.5 oz. M: 6 oz.	F: 31 M: 41	F: 143 M: 191	F: 1 M: 2	F: 0 M: 0	F: 0 M: 0
Tilapia, baked	F: 4 oz. M: 5 oz.	F: 30 M: 37	F: 145 M: 182	F: 3 M: 4	F: 1 M: 1	F: 0 M: 0
Tuna, canned in water	F: 4 oz. M: 6 oz.	F: 29 M: 43	F: 131 M: 197	F: 1 M: 1.5	F: 0 M: 0	F: 0 M: 0
Grouper, baked	F: 4.5 oz. M: 6 oz.	F: 31 M: 42	F: 150 M: 200	F: 2 M: 3	F: 0 M: 0.5	F: 0 M: 0
Chicken breast, white meat, boneless	F: 3 oz. M: 5 oz.	F: 27 M: 45	F: 138 M: 230	F: 3 M: 5	F: 0 M: 0	F: 0 M: 0
Turkey breast, roasted	F: 3.5 oz. M: 5 oz.	F: 30 M: 43	F: 133 M: 191	F: 1 M: 1	F: 0 M: 0	F: 0 M: 0
Turkey, white meat, roasted	F: 4 oz. M: 5 oz.	F: 33 M: 41	F: 215 M: 268	F: 8 M: 10	F: 2 M: 3	F: 0 M: 0
Ostrich, ground	F: 4 oz. M: 5 oz.	F: 30 M: 37	F: 199 M: 248	F: 8 M: 10	F: 2 M: 3	F: 0 M: 0
Turkey, dark meat, roasted	F: 4 oz. M: 5 oz.	F: 31 M: 39	F: 196 M: 245	F: 7 M: 9	F: 2 M: 3	F: 0 M: 0
Chicken breast, dark meat, boneless	F: 4 oz. M: 5 oz.	F: 31 M: 39	F: 232 M: 291	F: 11 M: 14	F: 3 M: 4	F: 0 M: 0
Duck breast, roasted	F: 4 oz. M: 6 oz.	F: 28 M: 42	F: 228 M: 342	F: 12 M: 18	F: 4 M: 6	F: 0 M: 0
Turkey leg	F: 4 oz. M: 5 oz.	F: 31 M: 40	F: 236 M: 295	F: 11 M: 14	F: 4 M: 4	F: 0 M: 0
Chicken thigh, boneless	F: 4 oz. M: 5 oz.	F: 28 M: 42	F: 280 M: 420	F: 17 M: 26	F: 5 M: 7	F: 0 M: 0

	Serving Size	Protein (g.)	Calories	Total Fat (g.)	Saturated Fat (g.)	Carbs (g.)
Bison, roasted	F: 4 oz. M: 5 oz.	F: 32 M: 40	F: 163 M: 203	F: 3 M: 4	F: 1 M: 1	F: 0 M: 0
Venison, broiled	F: 3.5 oz. M: 5 oz.	F: 30 M: 43	F: 149 M: 213	F: 2 M: 3	F: 1 M: 1	F: 0 M: 0
Pork tenderloin, roasted	F: 4 oz. M: 5 oz.	F: 30 M: 37	F: 163 M: 203	F: 4 M: 5	F: 1 M: 2	F: 0 M: 0
Eye round, lean, roasted	F: 3.5 oz. M: 5 oz.	F: 29 M: 41	F: 167 M: 238	F: 5 M: 7	F: 2 M: 3	F: 0 M: 0
Jerky (turkey)	1 oz.	15	80	0.5	0	3
Pork tenderloin, broiled	F: 3 oz. M: 4.5 oz.	F: 26 M: 39	F: 159 M: 239	F: 5 M: 8	F: 2 M: 3	F: 0 M: 0
Beef brisket, lean, braised	F: 3 oz. M: 4 oz.	F: 28 M: 38	F: 174 M: 232	F: 6 M: 8	F: 2 M: 3	F: 0 M: 0
Top sirloin steak, broiled	F: 3.5 oz. M: 5 oz.	F: 30 M: 43	F: 184 M: 263	F: 6 M: 9	F: 2 M: 3	F: 0 M: 0
Ground beef patty, 95% lean	F: 4 oz. M: 5 oz.	F: 30 M: 37	F: 193 M: 242	F: 7 M: 9	F: 3 M: 4	F: 0 M: 0
Bottom round, lean, roasted	F: 4 oz. M: 5 oz.	F: 31 M: 39	F: 200 M: 250	F: 7 M: 9	F: 3 M: 3	F: 0 M: 0
Filet mignon, lean, broiled	F: 3.5 oz. M: 5 oz.	F: 29 M: 41	F: 204 M: 292	F: 9 M: 13	F: 4 M: 5	F: 0 M: 0
Veal chop, lean, braised	F: 3 oz. M: 4 oz.	F: 29 M: 40	F: 192 M: 256	F: 8 M: 11	F: 2 M: 1	F: 0 M: 0
Flank steak, lean, broiled	F: 4 oz. M: 5 oz.	F: 31 M: 39	F: 220 M: 275	F: 9 M: 12	F: 4 M: 5	F: 0 M: 0
Beef tenderloin, lean, roasted	F: 4 oz. M: 5 oz.	F: 31 M: 39	F: 239 M: 298	F: 12 M: 15	F: 4 M: 6	F: 0 M: 0
Lamb chop, lean, broiled	F: 4 oz. M: 6 oz.	F: 28 M: 43	F: 208 M: 311	F: 9 M: 14	F: 3 M: 5	F: 0 M: 0
Top round steak, broiled	F: 3.5 oz. M: 5 oz.	F: 30 M: 43	F: 215 M: 307	F: 10 M: 14	F: 4 M: 5	F: 0 M: 0

	Serving Size	Protein (g.)	Calories	Total Fat (g.)	Saturated Fat (g.)	Carbs (g.)
Canadian bacon, grilled	1 slice	6	44	2	1	F: 0 M: 0
Chuck roast, blade, braised	F: 3 oz. M: 4.5 oz.	F: 26 M: 35	F: 213 M: 284	F: 11 M: 15	F: 4 M: 6	F: 0 M: 0
T-bone, lean, broiled	F: 4 oz. M: 6 oz.	F: 29 M: 44	F: 224 M: 336	F: 12 M: 16	F: 4 M: 6	F: 0 M: 0
Rib eye steak, lean, broiled	F: 3.5 oz. M: 5 oz.	F: 30 M: 43	F: 246 M: 352	F: 13 M: 19	F: 6 M: 8	F: 0 M: 0
Ground beef patty, 70% lean	F: 3 oz. M: 5 oz.	F: 22 M: 29	F: 239 M: 315	F: 15 M: 21	F: 6 M: 8	F: 0 M: 0
Flank steak, lean, braised	F: 3.5 oz. M: 5 oz.	F: 27 M: 38	F: 261 M: 373	F: 16 M: 23	F: 7 M: 10	F: 0 M: 0
Ground beef patty, 80% lean	F: 4 oz. M: 5 oz.	F: 27 M: 34	F: 279 M: 349	F: 18 M: 22	F: 7 M: 9	F: 0 M: 0
Bacon, regular	2 slices	5	69	5	2	F: 0 M: 0
Jerky (beef)	1 oz.	10	116	7	3	3

GROUP 2: HEALTHY FATS

It's hard to place healthy fats in the best order because, to be honest, each has its own unique added benefits. For example, cashews are excellent at triggering a serotonin release and for contributing to healthy brain function. Walnuts are specifically fantastic for testosterone production, making them an ideal choice for men.

That said, I want you to have five or six healthy fats in your quiver that are quick and easy go-to's for you to include in 25Days. But if weight loss is your main goal, I've arranged them by calories. By picking higher up on the chart, you'll be able to satisfy your fat-gram needs for whatever meal or snack you're building using foods that contain fewer calories.

One thing to note: when using olive oil (or any oil for that matter), try not to cook with it. What that does is agitate the molecular structure of the fats inside, which changes its value, and what was once a healthy fat becomes transformed into something less healthy for your body. So drizzle it instead of cooking in it if possible.

HEALTHY FATS

WOMEN: 10g. each meal/5g. each snack
MEN: 15g. each meal/7.5g. each snack

	Serving Size	Total Fat (g.)	Calories	Protein (g.)	Carbs (g.)	Saturated Fat (g.)
Olive oil	1 tsp.	5	40	0	0	1
Walnuts, raw	1 tbsp.	5	48	2	1	0
Brazil nuts, raw	¼ oz.	5	45	1	1	1
Pecans, raw	¼ oz.	5	50	1	1	0.5
Hazelnuts (or filberts), raw	¼ oz.	4.5	44	1	1	0
Macadamia nuts, raw	¼ oz.	5	50	0.5	1	1
Sunflower seeds, raw	1 tbsp.	5	51	2	2	0
Almond butter	½ tbsp.	4.5	51	1.5	1.5	0.5
Sesame seeds, roasted	1 tbsp.	5	52	2	2	0
Olives	14 (small)	5	53	0.5	2.5	0.5
Peanuts, raw	⅓ oz.	5	53	3	1.5	1
Flaxseeds, whole	1 tbsp.	4	55	2	3	0
Cashew butter	½ tbsp.	5	55	1.5	2.5	1
Avocado	¼ cup	5	58	1	3	1
Almonds, raw	⅓ oz.	5	63	2	2	1

	Serving Size	Total Fat (g.)	Calories	Protein (g.)	Carbs (g.)	Saturated Fat (g.)
Cashews, raw	½ oz.	6	83	2	5	1
Pumpkin seeds, roasted	1 oz.	5	125	5	15	1

GROUP 3: LOW-GLYCEMIC FIBROUS CARBOHYDRATES

Look at this chart, and I know what you're thinking. "Hey wait! It's in alphabetical order." Here's why: when I mentioned earlier in this chapter that you would be eating foods low on the glycemic index scale, high-fiber vegetables that cause a trickle of glucose in your system that keeps your sugar levels from spiking and prevents the release of insulin.

All of the vegetables (and the tomato, which is a fruit, by the way) fall below 40 on the glycemic index. That's the number I've always given clients to stay below to reduce insulin secretion. Most of the suggestions I've listed average 15 or less, and because each contains its own mixture of vitamins and minerals, it's the one I wouldn't dare put in any nutritional order—mostly because I want you to choose what you want to eat.

So if you're more inclined to eat broccoli than spinach, or you love snow peas more than eggplant, choose whatever you prefer. I want you to stick with the plan, so whichever of these makes that happen, they're the best choice for you.

LOW-GLYCEMIC FIBROUS CARBOHYDRATES

WOMEN: 20g. each meal/10g. each snack
MEN: 30g. each meal/15g. each snack

	GI Rating	Serving Size	Carbs (g.)	Calories	Protein (g.)	Total Fat (g.)
Artichoke	15	1 small	10	50	3	0
Asparagus	15	4 oz.	5	25	3	0

	GI Rating	Serving Size	Carbs (g.)	Calories	Protein (g.)	Total Fat (g.)
Bell pepper	15	½ cup	5	20	.5	0
Broccoli	15	¾ cup	5	22	2	0
Brussels sprouts	15	1 cup	11	56	4	1
Cabbage, chopped	15	1 cup	5	22	1	0
Carrot, raw	35	1 medium	6	25	.5	0
Cauliflower	15	1 cup	5	25	2	0
Celery	15	2 large stalks	4	20	0	0
Cucumber, peeled	15	1 8-inch	5	34	2	0
Eggplant	15	1 cup	9	35	1	0
Kale	15	½ cup	4	20	2	.5
Lettuce (Boston, iceberg, or romaine)	15	12 large leaves	4 to 5	20 to 23	1	0
Portabella mushroom	15	1 cup	4	22	2	0
Snap green beans	15	12	5	20	1	0
Snow peas, steamed	15	½ cup	6	35	2	0
Spinach, raw or cooked	15	5 oz.	5	33	4	0
Summer squash, baked	15	½ cup	11	41	1	0
Tomato	15	1 medium	5	22	1	0
Zucchini, steamed	15	¾ cup	5	21	1	0

GROUP 4: FRUITS

The reason I have this chart so far down the list is simple: if you're going to eat fruit, I want you to try limiting it to snacks only.

A lot of people tend to eat too much fruit because they see it as a fat-free food. But the fructose found in fruit, depending on where that fruit falls within the glycemic index, could also pull you out of what we're trying to accomplish, which is to utilize fat as energy. What I've done is to arrange some of my favorite fruits by where they rank on the glycemic index. If possible, try to pick options closer to the top of the list. But again, I want you to choose what you believe you'll stick to.

You'll also notice that a few of my free-for-all foods are on the list as well, such as apples, peaches, and cherries. I put those in for two reasons: first, so you can see where they fall among others nutritionally. And second, to make you aware that you're welcome to use those foods as part of your snack too, even though you're free to eat them all day long.

FRUITS						
	GI Rating	Serving Size	Carbs (g.)	Calories	Protein (g.)	Total Fat (g.)
Cherries (sour)	22	½ cup	9	39	1	0
Grapefruit	25	½ medium	10	41	1	0
Apricot, fresh	34	2 or 3	5	20	0	0
Apple	36	1 small	20	78	0	0
Pear	38	½ small	11	40	0	0
Plum	39	1 small	6	26	0	0
Blueberries	40	½ cup	11	41	1	0
Strawberries, whole	40	1 cup	11	46	1	0
Blackberries	40	4 oz.	11	49	1.5	.5
Peach	42	1 medium	9	38	1	0
Orange	45	1 small or ½ large	11	45	1	0

	GI Rating	Serving Size	Carbs (g.)	Calories	Protein (g.)	Total Fat (g.)
Banana	48	1 6-inch	20	72	1	0
Mango	51	2 oz.	10	40	0	0
Kiwi	53	1 medium	11	46	1	0
Papaya	58	⅔ cup	10	41	1	0
Pineapple	59	½ cup	10	37	0	0
Grapes (green or red)	59	10	9	34	1	0
Raisins (purple and seedless)	64	1 oz.	22	85	1	0
Honeydew	65	⅔ cup	10	41	1	0
Cantaloupe	65	¾ cup	10	41	1	0
Watermelon, diced	72	1 cup	11	45	1	0

GROUP 5: DAIRY

I'm personally not a big fan of milk, and as a rule, I don't typically recommend it to my clients either. Why? First and foremost, because of the excessive amount of hormones that are typically pumped into dairy cattle. But even if you choose milk options that are hormone free, there are a few other considerations you need to know about.

A lot of people worry about the fat content in milk. Fat, however, isn't the bad part in milk. It's lactose, the sugar found in milk, that's the bigger concern, because lactose causes a glycemic response, which negates the body's ability to utilize fat as energy. So even though milk is a great source of protein, its sugar content is enough to inhibit the changes we're trying to promote using 25Days.

Another reason is that I want you to eat your protein—not drink it. Liquids aren't digested but absorbed across the cell membrane, which prevents them from stoking your metabolism. As an absorbable, nonmetabolizing food, they skip the digestive process, so you burn fewer calories, whereas consuming a solid form of protein, such as eggs, fish, chicken, and so forth, forces your body to digest those foods and burn calories as a result.

So why didn't I leave out dairy entirely? Because I recognize that it might be one of the few options you have. It's also a protein source that has a biological value higher than the BVs for fish, chicken, beef, and pork. In fact, 90 percent of the protein you ingest is utilized immediately by your body, with only 10 percent left for waste.

DAIRY

	Serving Size	Protein (g.)	Calories	Total Fat (g.)	Saturated Fat (g.)	Carbs (g.)
Milk (nonfat)	10 oz.	10	100	1	0	14
Milk (1%)	10 oz.	10	138	3	2	16
Milk (2%)	10 oz.	10	154	6	4	14
Milk (whole)	10 oz.	10	185	10	6	15
Cottage cheese (nonfat)	3 oz.	9	600	0	6	
Kefir (plain low-fat)	1 cup	11	110	2	1.5	12
Goat milk	10 oz.	11	210	13	8	14
Goat cheese (soft)	1 oz.	5	76	6	4	0

GROUP 6: STARCHY CARBS

Even though all vegetables and fruits have a little starch in them, some are a lot richer than others. Those are the ones you'll find on this list. *They're also the ones you'll be eating only at the end of every block in your Every-Five-Day Mind Meal.*

For convenience, I've divided the chart into three types of starchy foods. I personally lean toward starchy vegetables, which is the reason I listed them first. However, I've included two other options as well. You'll find starchy breads and grains, as well as a few tried-and-true legumes. You can try the ones I've listed for convenience or pick any form of bread or legume, since no matter what shape, size, or color, you'll be eating a starchy carbohydrate. Also, if you're wondering why fruit isn't on the list, although there are a few starchy fruits, such as bananas, dried fruits, plantains, and figs, I prefer that you stick with these three options.

Finally, I've arranged them in no particular order, mostly because this is your reward. I'm letting you decide what works best for your body and whatever it's craving on that day. But don't worry: no matter which foods you choose, you'll still be resetting your hormone levels, lowering cortisol, replenishing serotonin, and restoring your glycogen levels.

STARCHY CARBS
STARCHY VEGETABLES

	GI Rating	Serving Size	Carbs (g.)	Calories	Protein (g.)	Total Fat (g.)
Beets, cooked	64	⅓ cup	6	24	1	0
Butternut squash, baked	51	½ cup	11	41	1	0
Corn, sweet yellow	55	⅓ cup	10	41	1	0
Peas	48	½ cup	10	59	4	4
Potato, baked with skin	85	1 small	30	128	3	0
Sweet potato, baked with skin or boiled	94 (baked) 46 (boiled)	1 small	12	54	1	0
Yams, cooked	54	¼ cup	9	39	1	0

STARCHY BREADS AND GRAINS

	GI Rating	Serving Size	Carbs (g.)	Calories	Protein (g.)	Total Fat (g.)
Bagel, plain	72	½ small	19	187	7	0
Bulgur, cooked	48	⅓ cup	11	50	2	0
Couscous, cooked	65	¼ cup	9	44	2	0
Ezekiel sprouted grain bread	36	1 slice	15	80	4	1
Pasta	43 to 61	1 oz.	20 (on average)	105 (on average)	4	1
Pita, whole wheat or white	68	½	17	84	3	0
Pumpernickel	46	½ slice	6	32	1	0
Quinoa, cooked	53	⅓ cup	20	108	4	1
Rice, basmati	52	¼ cup	10	50	1	0
Rice, brown	55	¼ cup	10	50	1	0
Rice, white, short-grain, or long-grain	79 (white) 72 (short) 56 (long)	¼ cup	13	61	1	0
Rye bread	41 to 55	1 slice	15	82	3	1
White, whole wheat, or seven-grain bread	70 to 75	½ slice	6 to 7	32 to 37	1	0

STARCHY LEGUMES						
	GI Rating	Serving Size	Carbs (g.)	Calories	Protein (g.)	Total Fat (g.)
Black beans	30	½ cup	20	114	8	0
Chickpeas (garbanzo beans)	38	⅔ cup	30	180	10	2
Kidney beans	29	½ cup	20	113	8	0
Lentils, boiled	29	½ cup	19	113	9	0

chapter six

The 25Days Recipes

he flexibility of the 25Days Diet makes it easy to mix and match foods to create any number of meals or snacks. But the genius of the program is that there isn't a limit to what you can prepare, so long as you stay within the nutritional requirements. To prove that point, I called upon the brilliance of the person who makes all of my meals— both for myself and the ones I count on when using 25Days with all of my celebrity clients—executive chef Jennifer Jewett.

In addition to having worked at some of the top restaurants in Los Angeles, she's the founder of First Spoonful, a meal delivery company specializing in healthy cuisine. Jennifer's clientele includes some of LA's most successful CEOs, celebrities, and professional athletes—and they all expect the best—something she has always been able to do with incredible ease. Personally, I believe that *you* expect the best as well, which is exactly why I brought her on board to help create twenty-five recipes for 25Days.

The first thing you may notice is that unlike the minimalist approach traditionally found in most diet and lifestyle books, a few of the 25Days recipes are a little longer—either regarding the number of ingredients or the number of steps involved to prepare them. But I have news for you: those extra ingredients and effort also mean a lot more taste and satisfaction, both of which will make it even easier to form a new neurological pattern and enjoy the program for life. And don't worry, because they're a lot easier to follow than you think. Even if you have zero experience in the kitchen, the twenty-five recipes aren't just doable—they're delicious.

Remember to Make It Fun

It's easy to make fitness a grueling and awful process that feels like work. But I don't do it because it feels like work, and neither do my clients. We do it because we genuinely enjoy it. So if you don't enjoy something, you have to question its approach.

The whole premise of 25Days is to form new neurological patterns by creating positive feelings and positive reinforcement around the healthy things that you're doing. If you love to cook, then you're naturally going to enjoy experimenting with the 25Days recipes, which will help retrain your brain. That being said, if you're looking at these recipes and thinking to yourself, "Oh! There's quite a bit of preparation involved, and I'm not sure I can do this," then here's what I want you to do:

Take a weekend, grab a few friends, pick a few recipes that you'll all enjoy—the ones that genuinely sound good to you—and make it a party by getting together and cooking. Turn it into an enjoyable social experience so that it instantly becomes part of your process. Besides, the way a few of the recipes are structured, you're going to have plenty of healthy leftovers to stick in the fridge for the next day, freeze for later in the week, or box up and share with others—so the more, the merrier.

To really boost that sense of positive reinforcement, try inviting friends who may be considering doing the program side by side with you. Or ask a few friends who don't think they can live a healthy lifestyle or who think that eating healthy is boring or never tastes good. Look at this moment as your chance not only to create an enjoyable experience but also to inspire someone else to change his or her life. Now let's get cooking!

Spinach and Pepper Baked Egg Casserole

Servings: 4

1 teaspoon olive oil
1 cup finely diced bell pepper
½ cup finely diced onion
Salt and pepper
2 tablespoons minced garlic
3 bunches fresh spinach, washed
   and chopped (about 4½ cups)

9 eggs
½ cup whole milk
1 ounce goat cheese, crumbled
¼ cup minced scallions
1 tablespoon minced basil
2 tablespoons minced parsley

Preheat oven to 325°F.

Heat a sauté pan on the stove top over medium heat. Add ½ teaspoon of the olive oil and sauté the bell pepper and onion until lightly browned and soft. Season with salt and pepper to taste and add the garlic and sauté for 1 minute. Remove the peppers and onions from the pan and place them in a bowl. In the same pan add the remaining ½ teaspoon olive oil and add the spinach 1 handful at a time. Sauté until the spinach has wilted, season with salt and pepper to taste, and place in a bowl lined with paper towels. Let drain for a couple of minutes, and then use the paper towels to squeeze out the rest of the liquid. Add the spinach to the bowl with the peppers and onions.

Whisk the eggs, milk, half the goat cheese, scallions, basil, parsley, and salt and pepper to taste until just combined. Add the vegetables. Coat a 9-x-9-inch baking dish with cooking spray and pour in the egg and vegetable mixture. Top with the rest of the crumbled goat cheese.

Place in the oven, uncovered, for 30 to 35 minutes until the casserole is completely set.

To serve: cut the casserole into 4 equal servings.

Per serving: 240 calories, 15 g. fat, 18 g. protein, 7 g. carbohydrates

Snap Pea and Zucchini Frittata with Roasted Cherry Tomatoes

Servings: 4

1½ teaspoons olive oil
½ cup finely diced zucchini
½ cup finely chopped snow peas
2 tablespoons minced shallots
Salt and pepper
1 tablespoon minced garlic

3 cups cherry tomatoes
8 eggs
½ cup whole milk
½ ounce grated Manchego cheese
¼ cup minced scallions
1 tablespoon minced basil

Preheat oven to 350°F.

Heat a 9-inch ovenproof sauté pan on the stove top over medium heat. Add ½ teaspoon olive oil and sauté the zucchini, snow peas, and shallots until they are lightly browned and soft. Season with salt and pepper to taste, and add the garlic and sauté for 1 more minute. Set aside.

Coat the cherry tomatoes with 1 teaspoon olive oil, season with salt and pepper to taste, and roast in the oven for about 15 minutes until blistered and soft. Halfway through the cooking time, shake the tomatoes and turn the baking sheet. Remove and set aside covered to keep warm.

Whisk the eggs, milk, cheese, scallions, basil, salt, and pepper until just combined. Do not overmix, or the frittata will be flat instead of fluffy. Heat the sautéed vegetables in the same pan until they begin to sizzle. Pour in the egg mixture and cook for 4 to 5 minutes, until the eggs begin to set. Place the whole pan in the oven and bake for 12 to 15 minutes, making sure the frittata is set. Once done, take out of the oven and let sit in the pan for 2 to 3 minutes.

To serve: gently slide the frittata out of the pan and cut into 8 wedges. Serve 2 slices of frittata with ¼ of the roasted cherry tomatoes.

Per serving: 227 calories, 14 g. fat, 15 g. protein, 8 g. carbohydrates

breakfast

DREW LOGAN

76

Chocolate Banana Muffins with Blueberry Butter

Servings: 18

Chocolate Banana Muffins

½ cup buckwheat flour
¾ cup coconut flour
1 cup almond flour
6 tablespoons cocoa powder
2 teaspoons baking powder
1 teaspoon baking soda
¼ teaspoon salt
½ cup coconut sugar

2 eggs
¼ cup coconut oil, melted
½ cup Greek yogurt
1 teaspoon vanilla extract
1 cup bananas, mashed
½ cup unsweetened applesauce
½ cup almond milk
Cooking spray

Blueberry Butter

1 pint blueberries
¼ cup water

1 tablespoon coconut sugar
1½ tablespoons coconut oil

MAKE THE MUFFINS:

Preheat oven to 350°F. In a large bowl, sift together the buckwheat flour, coconut flour, almond flour, cocoa powder, baking powder, baking soda, salt, and coconut sugar.

In another large bowl, whisk together the eggs, coconut oil, yogurt, vanilla, bananas, applesauce, and almond milk.

Add the dry ingredients to the wet ingredients and mix well.

Coat a mini muffin pan with cooking spray and scoop out batter for 36 muffins. You will have to bake the muffins in 2 batches. The batter is dense, so you can form them into balls and press them gently into the muffin tin.

Bake for 10 minutes, and then rotate the pan and bake for another 10 minutes. Let sit for 5 minutes in the pan and then remove them.

MAKE THE BLUEBERRY BUTTER:

Cook the blueberries in a small pan with the water and coconut sugar for about 10 minutes. Pour the mixture into a high-powered blender with the coconut oil and puree well until an emulsified butter is formed. Divide the butter into 12 servings.

To serve: each serving consists of 2 mini muffins. Serve the muffins warm with 1 serving of the blueberry butter. Warm any leftover muffins before serving.

Per serving: 162 calories, 9 g. fat, 4 g. protein, 19 g. carbohydrates

Chicken Sausage Patties

Servings: 8

1 pound lean ground chicken
¼ teaspoon onion powder
¼ teaspoon garlic powder
¼ teaspoon ground coriander
¼ teaspoon ground cumin
¼ teaspoon ground fennel

¼ teaspoon minced fresh thyme
¼ teaspoon minced fresh rosemary
½ teaspoon coconut sugar
½ teaspoon salt
¼ teaspoon pepper
1 teaspoon olive oil

Preheat oven to 350°F.

Mix together the chicken, onion and garlic powder, coriander, cumin, fennel, thyme, rosemary, coconut sugar, salt, and pepper and cover with plastic wrap. Let sit in the refrigerator for at least 1 hour to marry the ingredients.

Divide into eight 2-ounce patties.

Heat an ovenproof sauté pan on the stove top on medium-high heat. Add the olive oil and place 4 of the patties in the pan. Cook on one side about 3 minutes until nice and golden, flip, and then immediately place the pan in the oven for another 4 minutes.

To serve: use as a side dish to any of the egg breakfasts.

Per serving: 86 calories, 1.5 g. fat, 15 g. protein, 0.5 g. carbohydrates

Zucchini, Spinach, Asparagus, and Goat Cheese Omelet

Servings: 4

¾ tablespoon olive oil

1 cup zucchini, cut into half moons

Salt and pepper

Dozen eggs

3 tablespoons water

¼ cup minced scallions

6 peeled asparagus spears

2 cups fresh spinach leaves

1 ounce goat cheese, crumbled

Heat a 9-inch sauté pan on the stove top over medium heat. Add ½ teaspoon olive oil and sauté the zucchini until it is lightly browned and soft. Season with salt and pepper to taste. Set aside.

Whisk together the eggs, water, scallions, and salt and pepper to taste to incorporate air into the egg mixture. Heat the same pan over medium heat, and add ¼ teaspoon of olive oil. Pour in the egg mixture and cook for 1 to 2 minutes, until the eggs begin to set. Add ¼ of the sautéed zucchini to one side of the pan and top it with ¼ of the asparagus and ¼ of the spinach leaves. Add ¼ ounce of the goat cheese to the top of the vegetables.

Use a rubber spatula to begin lifting the outer edges of the omelet. Once the edges are coming up easily and most of the egg is fully cooked, fold the omelet in half. Let cook another minute and gently slide out of the pan.

Cook the remaining omelets. These can be refrigerated and heated up for the next three mornings.

To serve: slide the omelets onto plates and enjoy.

Per serving: 263 calories, 18 g. fat, 20 g. protein, 2 g. carbohydrates

Spinach and Blueberry Protein Shake

Servings: 4

Almond Milk

2 cups whole almonds

4 cups filtered water and more if necessary

Shake

2 cups spinach

1 cup roughly chopped kale, leaves only

¾ cup frozen blueberries

1½ cups almond milk

1½ cups coconut water

½ banana

2 scoops unflavored Garden of Life protein powder

Zest and juice of 1 lemon

1 tablespoon chia seeds

1 tablespoon maca root powder

1 tablespoon bee pollen

¼ teaspoon turmeric

8 drops schisandra berry liquid

MAKE THE ALMOND MILK:

Cover the 2 cups of almonds with water. Let sit overnight. In the morning, rinse the almonds well and puree them in a high-powered blender. Pour in the 4 cups of filtered water. Blend for 5 minutes, starting on low and gradually moving to high. Pour the mixture into a nut bag that is sitting in a large glass bowl. Strain the nut mixture, gently squeezing the bag to make sure you get all the almond milk. I always add about 1 cup of the almond meal that is left over in the bag back into the almond milk; it gives a nice, thick texture and adds a lot of the protein back into the milk.

This makes about 4 cups of almond milk. Take out 1½ cups for this recipe. Place the rest in a covered glass container and refrigerate. Almond milk will keep in your refrigerator about three days.

MAKE THE SHAKE:

In a high-powered blender, combine the spinach, kale, blueberries, almond milk, coconut water, banana, protein powder, lemon zest and juice, chia seeds, maca root powder, bee pollen, turmeric, and schisandra berry liquid.

Blend until the ingredients are well combined and of a smoothie consistency.

To serve: pour into four glasses.

Per serving: 195 calories, 9.6 g. fat, 17 g. protein, 15.5 g. carbohydrates

Grilled Shrimp Salad with Zucchini Ribbons and Toasted Almond Pesto

Servings: 3

Shrimp

½ pound wild shrimp, peeled and deveined
¼ teaspoon olive oil

¼ teaspoon smoked paprika
Salt and pepper

Toasted Almond Pesto

½ cup toasted almonds
2 cloves garlic
1 teaspoon salt
Zest and juice of 1 lemon
½ cup fresh basil leaves

¼ cup fresh cilantro leaves
¼ cup fresh parsley leaves
¼ cup fresh tarragon leaves
1 tablespoon olive oil
Water as needed

Salad

4 cups spinach, washed and dried
4 cups mixed greens, washed and dried
½ cup thinly sliced cucumber

1 zucchini, cut into ribbons (use either a spiralizer or a mandoline with the julienne attachment)
½ cup cherry tomatoes, halved

PREPARE THE SHRIMP:

Coat the shrimp in the olive oil, paprika, and salt and pepper to taste. Heat a grill pan on medium until it's smoking. Add the shrimp and grill, let sit for 3 minutes until they begin to turn opaque. Flip the shrimp and grill on the other side until completely cooked. This will take about 6 minutes.

MAKE THE PESTO:

Put the almonds, garlic, salt, lemon zest and juice, and all the herbs into a blender. Turn on the blender and slowly add the olive oil. Add water as needed to loosen the mixture and allow it to blend until a loose pesto is formed. Should make about 1 cup.

To serve: combine the spinach and mixed greens, then place ⅓ of the greens in three separate bowls. Top each salad with ⅓ of the cucumbers, ⅓ of the zucchini ribbons, ⅓ of the cherry tomatoes, and 3 ounces of the grilled shrimp. Use about 3.5 ounces of pesto per salad.

Per serving: 249 calories, 14 g. fat, 21 g. protein, 10 g. carbohydrates

Greek Salad with Oregano Grilled Chicken and Cashew Tzatziki Dressing

Servings: 4

Chicken

1 cup bell pepper, cut into strips

2 teaspoons olive oil

Salt and pepper

1 pound boneless, skinless chicken breasts, pounded

½ teaspoon smoked paprika

1 tablespoon dried oregano

Cashew Tzatziki Dressing

2 tablespoons minced dill

1 cup watercress

½ cup cashews

1 cup cucumber

3 garlic cloves, minced

Zest and juice of 2 lemons

Salad

1 tablespoon minced parsley

1 tablespoon minced dill sprigs

1 tablespoon minced mint

4 tablespoons chopped Kalamata olives

1 cup thinly sliced cucumber

1 cup cherry tomatoes, halved lengthwise

1 cup watercress

4 cups arugula

4 cups spinach

½ cup minced scallions

Zest of 1 lemon

Preheat oven to 350°F.

PREPARE THE CHICKEN:

Coat the bell pepper strips in ½ teaspoon olive oil, and salt and pepper to taste, and roast in the oven for about 10 minutes until soft. Dice finely and set aside.

Heat a grill pan until smoking; then turn it down to medium. Coat the chicken in the remaining olive oil, paprika, oregano, and salt and pepper to taste. Grill on one side for about 6 minutes until nice grill marks have formed and the chicken is ¾ of the way cooked. Flip the chicken and grill on the other side to cook through. Set aside.

MAKE THE DRESSING:

Place the dill, watercress, cashews, cucumber, garlic, and lemon zest and juice in a high-powered blender and blend until all ingredients are combined.

In a large bowl, combine the parsley, dill, mint, olives, roasted bell peppers, cucumber, cherry tomatoes, watercress, arugula, spinach, scallions, and lemon zest. Toss everything together. Plate into 4 servings.

To serve: cut the chicken into strips and divide into 4 portions. Top each salad with ¼ of the chicken. Serve each salad with ¼ cup of dressing.

Per serving: 338 calories, 15.5 g. fat, 32 g. protein, 13.5 g. carbohydrates

Za'tar Roasted Chicken Cabbage Cups

Servings: 6

Filling

1 tablespoon dried oregano

1 tablespoon dried thyme

1 tablespoon sumac

1 tablespoon sesame
    seeds

Salt and pepper

12 ounces boneless, skinless
    chicken breasts, cut into me-
    dium dice

1 head purple cabbage

Cooking spray

4 tablespoons chopped green olives

1 cup thinly sliced cucumber

½ cup finely diced avocado

¼ cup sunflower sprouts

Lemon Tahini Dressing

½ cup tahini

1 tablespoon minced parsley

3 garlic cloves, minced

5 dashes hot sauce

Zest and juice of 4 lemons

3 tablespoons olive oil

1 teaspoon salt

Preheat oven to 350°F.

MAKE THE FILLING:

Combine the oregano, thyme, sumac, sesame seeds, and salt and pepper to taste. Toss the chicken in about 2 tablespoons of the spice mixture; reserve the rest of the spice mixture.

Cut off the bottom root of the purple cabbage and gently remove the leaves. Try to keep the leaves whole so that they remain looking like cups. Set aside.

Coat a baking sheet generously with cooking spray and place the chicken on top. Bake for about 6 minutes until the chicken is cooked all the way through; turn halfway through. Take out and set aside.

Put the olives, cucumber, avocado, and sunflower sprouts into a bowl and toss with a teaspoon of the reserved spice mixture. Taste and add more spice mixture if needed. Add the diced chicken and toss all ingredients together. Set aside.

MAKE THE DRESSING:
Combine the tahini, parsley, garlic, hot sauce, lemon zest and juice, olive oil, and salt,

To serve: lay out 6 of the cabbage cups and scoop the chicken mixture evenly into each. Each serving is 1 cabbage cup. Serve with 2 ounces of lemon tahini dressing on the side.

Per serving: 355 calories, 24 g. fat, 20 g. protein, 7 g. carbohydrates

Tarragon Shrimp Salad

Servings: 4

Shrimp

1 pound shrimp, deveined, shells on

8 cups water

2 sprigs tarragon

1 tablespoon whole dill sprigs

1 cup roughly chopped tomatoes

1 teaspoon white peppercorns

2 bay leaves

1 lemon, sliced

Salad

1 tablespoon minced dill sprigs

1 tablespoon minced tarragon

1 cup finely diced tomatoes

1 cup finely diced cucumber

2 celery stalks, minced

1 finely diced bell pepper

6 scallions, minced

1 garlic clove, minced

Zest and juice of 1 lemon

2 tablespoons minced shallots

2 tablespoons olive oil

Salt and pepper to taste

PREPARE THE SHRIMP:

Remove the shells from the shrimp and place the shells in a large saucepan. Top with the water, and add the tarragon, dill, tomatoes, peppercorns, bay leaves, and lemon. Bring to a boil and simmer for about 30 minutes. Turn down to a low simmer and drop the shrimp into the poaching liquid. Stir. Cook for about 3 minutes and then turn off the heat. Let the shrimp sit in the liquid for another 2 minutes. Strain the liquid (you can keep it to use again for up to three days), remove the shrimp, place in the refrigerator, and let cool completely.

Toss together all the salad ingredients; let marinate for about an hour. Remove the shrimp from the refrigerator and chop into bite-sized pieces.

To serve: toss the shrimp with the salad ingredients and divide into 4 servings. Can be served as is or over mixed greens.

Per serving: 215 calories, 9 g. fat, 24 g. protein, 9 g. carbohydrates

Greek Chicken Swiss Chard Wrap with Garlic Yogurt Dressing

Servings: 4

Chicken

12 ounces boneless, skinless chicken breasts, cut into medium dice
¼ teaspoon dried oregano
1 tablespoon minced parsley

1 tablespoon minced dill
¼ teaspoon smoked paprika
Salt and pepper
Cooking spray

Garlic Yogurt Dressing

1 cup Greek yogurt
1 tablespoon minced dill
1 tablespoon minced parsley

3 garlic cloves, minced
5 dashes hot sauce
Zest and juice of 1 lemon

Wrap

1 cup finely diced tomato
4 tablespoons chopped olives
1 cup finely diced bell peppers
1 cup thinly sliced cucumber
½ cup finely diced avocado

½ cup feta cheese, crumbled
1 cup mixed greens
4 leaves Swiss chard, center stem removed, washed and dried

Preheat oven to 350°F.

PREPARE THE CHICKEN:

Sprinkle the chicken pieces with the oregano, parsley, dill, paprika, and salt and pepper to taste. Coat a baking sheet generously with cooking spray and place the chicken on top. Bake for about 6 minutes until the chicken is cooked all the way through; turn halfway through. Take out of the oven and set aside.

MAKE THE YOGURT DRESSING:

Combine the yogurt, dill, parsley, garlic, hot sauce, and lemon zest and juice. Stir, and set aside.

Put the tomato, olives, bell peppers, cucumber, avocado, feta, and mixed greens into a bowl and toss with 8 tablespoons of the yogurt dressing.

To serve: lay out each Swiss chard leaf vertically and fold the bottoms over one another so the leaf is one piece. Divide the tomato mixture into 4 and lay on top of the Swiss chard. Lay ¼ of the chicken on top of each vegetable pile. Wrap the Swiss chard like a burrito and cut in half.

Per serving: 225 calories, 9 g. fat, 25 g. protein, 8 g. carbohydrates

Stuffed Bell Peppers with Ground Chicken, Tomatoes, and Zucchini

Servings: 4

½ tablespoon olive oil
½ cup minced onion
1 cup finely diced zucchini
Salt and pepper
3 cloves garlic, minced
1 tablespoon tomato paste
1½ pounds ground white meat
  chicken

14.5-ounce can crushed
  tomatoes
½ cup chicken stock
¼ cup minced basil
¼ cup minced parsley
4 bell peppers, tops cut off, cores
  and seeds removed
Cooking spray

Preheat oven to 350°F.

Heat a small sauté pan over medium heat, and add the olive oil. Add the onion and zucchini and sauté until they are soft. Then add salt and pepper to taste, add the garlic, and sauté for 1 more minute. Add the tomato paste and stir to combine.

Add the ground chicken and break apart the meat; season again with salt and pepper. Pour in the tomatoes and stir. Let cook for 20 minutes. Add the chicken stock, basil, and parsley, stir, and let reduce for about 8 minutes.

Coat a small casserole dish with cooking spray, place the bell peppers in the dish. Spray the inside of them with cooking spray and season them with salt and pepper. Scoop the chicken and vegetable mixture evenly into the bell peppers. Cover with foil and bake for 20 minutes.

To serve: one bell pepper is a serving. Enjoy!

Per serving: 253.5 calories, 15.25 g. fat, 33 g. protein, 15 g. carbohydrates

Salmon Cakes with Yogurt Tartar Sauce and Grilled Peppers and Fennel

Servings: 4

Salmon Cakes

¾ pound boneless wild salmon fillet, skin on
2 teaspoons olive oil
Salt and pepper
1 cup finely diced yellow bell peppers
¼ cup finely diced onion
1 cup finely diced cremini mushrooms
1 clove garlic, minced

1 tablespoon minced parsley
2 teaspoons Dijon mustard
1 scallion, minced
1 tablespoon Worcestershire sauce
¼ teaspoon Old Bay seasoning
Zest of 1 lemon
1 egg
¼ cup almond flour
½ tablespoon minced dill
Cooking spray

Yogurt Tartar Sauce

½ cup Greek yogurt
1½ teaspoons Dijon mustard
3 dashes Worcestershire sauce
Juice of 1 lemon

2 cornichons (pickled gherkins), minced
1 teaspoon minced capers
¼ teaspoon mustard powder
5 dashes hot sauce
1 tablespoon minced parsley

Grilled Bell Peppers and Fennel

3 yellow bell peppers, skinned and seeded and cut into 4 pieces
1 fennel bulb, sliced lengthwise in 1-inch strips

1 teaspoon olive oil
Salt and pepper

Preheat oven to 350°F.

MAKE THE SALMON CAKES:
Place the salmon fillet, skin side down, on a sheet tray, drizzle with 1 teaspoon of olive oil, and season with salt and pepper to taste. Put into

the oven and bake for 7 minutes. The salmon should be medium to medium rare. Set aside.

Sauté the bell peppers, onion, and mushrooms in 1 teaspoon of olive oil, and season with salt and pepper. Sauté until softened and starting to brown, add the garlic, and sauté for another minute. Place the softened vegetables into a large mixing bowl.

Add the parsley, mustard, scallion, Worcestershire sauce, Old Bay seasoning, lemon zest, and egg to the sautéed vegetables. Stir together all the ingredients to combine. Season with salt and pepper. Remove the salmon fillet from the skin and gently pull apart the salmon to flake it. Combine it with the vegetables. Add the almond flour, dill, and salt and pepper to taste; mix everything together gently. You want to keep the salmon in larger flakes so that the salmon cakes remain tender.

Scoop into ¼-cup-sized patties and form into round balls. Spray a plate with a little cooking spray and place the patties on the plate, cover with plastic wrap, and place in the refrigerator for 30 minutes to set up.

Preheat oven to 400°F.

MAKE THE YOGURT TARTAR SAUCE:
Combine the yogurt, mustard, Worcestershire sauce, lemon juice, cornichons, capers, mustard powder, hot sauce, and parsley in a bowl and stir. Set aside.

MAKE THE GRILLED BELL PEPPERS AND FENNEL:
Season the peppers and fennel with olive oil, and salt and pepper to taste. Heat a grill pan over medium-high heat until the pan is smoking. Place the vegetables on the grill pan and cook for 4 minutes on one side until brown grill marks form. Flip the vegetables over and continue cooking until they are soft. Remove from pan and set aside. Cover with foil to keep warm.

Spray a sheet tray with cooking spray, place the 8 salmon cakes on it, place in the oven, and cook for 10 to 12 minutes.

To serve: place 2 salmon cakes on each plate with 2 tablespoons of the yogurt tartar sauce, divide the grilled vegetables into 4 equal servings, and serve 1 each with 2 salmon cakes.

Per serving: 296 calories, 15 g. fat, 24 g. protein, 14.5 g. carbohydrates

Chicken Milanese with Green Apple and Watercress Salad

Servings: 4

Chicken

½ cup almond flour

3 tablespoons grated Parmesan cheese

2 tablespoons minced parsley

1 teaspoon minced fresh oregano

1 tablespoon minced fresh sage

1 teaspoon minced fresh thyme

Salt and pepper

2 eggs

2 tablespoons water

1 pound boneless, skinless chicken breast, pounded and cut into 4 pieces

Cooking spray

Salad

2 bunches watercress, roots cut off, washed

2 cups arugula

1 cup finely diced green apple, cored

1 shallot, medium, minced

Zest and juice of 2 lemons

Preheat oven to 375°F.

PREPARE THE CHICKEN:

In a bowl, place the almond flour, Parmesan cheese, 1 tablespoon parsley, ½ teaspoon oregano, ½ tablespoon sage, all the thyme, and a little salt and pepper, and stir to combine. In another bowl, whisk the eggs with the water and a little salt and pepper.

Coat a sheet tray with cooking spray. Place each chicken breast in the egg mixture, let the excess drip off, and coat it well in the almond flour mixture. Place each chicken breast on the prepared sheet tray. Bake for about 10 minutes until the chicken is cooked through and the almond flour is lightly browned.

MAKE THE SALAD:

In a large bowl, combine the watercress, arugula, apple, shallot, the remainder of the herbs, and a little salt and pepper. Set aside.

To serve: toss the salad with the lemon juice right before serving. Place one chicken breast on each plate and top with ¼ of the salad mixture.

Per serving: 275 calories, 12 g. fat, 34 g. protein, 7 g. carbohydrates

Grilled Chicken with Harissa Zucchini Falafel Salad, Cashew Tzatziki, and Pickled Beets

Servings: 8

Pickled Beets

2 medium-sized red beets	1 cup of water
Olive oil	½ cup red wine vinegar
Salt and pepper	1 tablespoon coconut sugar

Falafel

3 cups zucchini, grated and squeezed dry	1 tablespoon harissa paste
¼ cup onion, grated	1 tablespoon flaxseeds
1 teaspoon tahini	1 egg
1 tablespoon parsley, minced	¼ cup coconut flour
½ teaspoon cumin	Salt and pepper
1 teaspoon baking powder	Cooking spray

Cashew Tzatziki

1 cup cashews	Zest and juice of 1 lemon
½ cup chopped cucumber	2 cloves garlic, minced
1 cup watercress	Salt and pepper
1 tablespoon dill	

Grilled Chicken

24 ounces skinless, boneless chicken breasts, pounded	Salt and pepper
1 tablespoon olive oil	1 tablespoon harissa paste

Preheat oven to 375°F.

PREPARE THE BEETS:

Rub the beets with a little olive oil and season with salt and pepper to taste. Place them in a loaf pan and pour in the water. Cover them with foil and bake for 45 minutes. Check them about a half hour in to make sure there is still water in the pan; if it has evaporated, add more. The beets are done when you can insert a paring knife into them easily without any resistance. Let cool for about 10 minutes.

Peel the skin off the beets and slice them into ¼-inch slices. Mix the vinegar, coconut sugar, and salt and pepper to taste in a small bowl and combine the mixture with the beet slices. Let it sit out for at least 1 hour. You can cook the beets up to two days in advance and leave them in the refrigerator covered; they will continue to taste better the longer they sit.

MAKE THE FALAFEL:

In a large bowl, combine the zucchini, onion, tahini, parsley, cumin, baking powder, harissa paste, flaxseeds, and egg. Stir well to combine and let sit for about 30 minutes. A lot of liquid will release from the zucchini and onion. After the 30 minutes, pour off the excess liquid, press the mixture gently to remove some more of the liquid, and drain it off. Add the coconut flour and salt and pepper to taste.

Form this mixture into eight equal-sized patties. Generously coat a sheet tray with cooking spray and place the patties on the sheet tray. Bake for 7 minutes on one side. Take the tray out of the oven. Flip the patties over carefully, return tray to oven, and bake for another 5 minutes.

MAKE THE TZATZIKI:

Place the cashews, cucumber, watercress, dill, lemon zest and juice, garlic, and salt and pepper to taste into a high-powered blender and blend until well combined.

PREPARE THE CHICKEN:

Cut the pounded breasts into eight 3-ounce portions. Heat a grill pan to high. Coat the chicken with the olive oil, salt and pepper to taste, and harissa paste. Lay the chicken on the grill pan and cook for about 6 minutes on one side. It's ready to flip when the chicken comes off the grill easily. Flip the chicken and cook for about another 3 minutes.

To serve: serve a 3-ounce grilled chicken breast with a scoop of falafel, 2 ounces of the tzatziki, and ⅛ of the pickled beet slices.

Per serving: 289 calories, 13.7 g. fat, 25 g. protein, 14 g. carbohydrates

Grilled Lemon Shrimp Bowl with Cauliflower Rice, Roasted Chili Broccoli, and Bell Peppers

Servings: 2

Roasted Chili Broccoli and Bell Peppers

1 cup broccoli florets
1 red bell pepper, cut into thin strips
½ tablespoon olive oil
Salt and pepper
¼ teaspoon red pepper flakes
Cooking spray

Grilled Lemon Shrimp Bowl

½ pound shrimp, peeled and deveined
½ tablespoon olive oil
2 cloves garlic, minced
Zest and juice of 2 lemons
Salt and pepper
2 tablespoons soy sauce
1 tablespoon sambal
2 cups cauliflower, blanched and riced
2 tablespoons scallions, minced
2 tablespoons pickled ginger (a good-quality store-bought brand)

Preheat oven to 350°F.

Toss the broccoli and bell pepper with olive oil, salt and pepper, and red pepper flakes. Coat a baking sheet with cooking spray and place the vegetables in the oven to roast for about 18 to 20 minutes.

Heat a grill pan over medium-high heat. Toss the shrimp with the olive oil, garlic, lemon zest and juice, and salt and pepper to taste. Grill the shrimp about 2 minutes on each side until fully cooked. Once cooked, toss with ½ of the soy sauce and ½ of the sambal.

To serve: stir the remaining soy sauce and sambal into the cauliflower rice and scoop out the rice into two bowls. Divide the roasted broccoli and pepper in half and place on top of the rice. Divide the shrimp in half and place on top of the vegetables. Top each bowl with ½ of the scallions and ½ of the pickled ginger.

Per serving: 246 calories, 7.75 g. fat, 27.5 g. protein, 11.75 g. carbohydrates

Spicy Mexican Shepherd's Pie

Servings: 6

2 heads cauliflower florets
Salt and pepper
3 tablespoons grated Parmesan
   cheese
2 poblano peppers
2 tablespoons olive oil
1 cup finely diced zucchini
1 cup finely diced onion
1 tablespoon seeded minced jalapeño pepper
2 cloves garlic, minced

3 tablespoons tomato paste
1½ pounds ground turkey
1 teaspoon coriander
½ teaspoon cumin
1½ teaspoons chili powder
½ cup chicken stock
1 teaspoon minced cilantro
1 sprig fresh thyme
1 cup sliced avocado
Cooking spray

Preheat oven to 375°F.

Bring a large pot of water to a boil. Add the cauliflower florets and cook until soft, about 10 minutes. Drain well and place in either a food processor or a high-speed blender and puree. Season with a little salt and pepper, add the Parmesan cheese, and mix. Set aside.

Turn on one of your stove top burners and place both poblanos over the open flame. Let them brown and char on all sides, using tongs to flip them over. Once completely charred, place them in a bowl and cover with plastic wrap for 10 minutes. Take out the peppers, peel off the charred skin, and discard it. Remove the tops of the poblanos, cut them open, and throw away all the seeds. Dice the poblanos.

Heat a large skillet over medium-high heat. Add the olive oil. Sauté the zucchini, onion, and jalapeño for about 5 minutes, until they are softened and beginning to brown. Add the garlic and sauté for 1 minute. Add the tomato paste and combine well with the vegetables.

Add the ground turkey, and break it up with a spatula, and cook for about 3 minutes, until the turkey begins to turn white. Add the coriander, cumin, chili powder, and a little salt and pepper to taste. Stir to combine. Add the chicken stock and scrape up all the browned bits from the pan. Take off the heat. Add the poblano peppers, cilantro, and thyme and stir to combine.

Spray a deep 9-inch ovenproof skillet with a little cooking spray and pour in the ground turkey mixture. Spread it evenly in the pan. Top with the cauliflower puree and spread it in an even layer over the turkey mixture.

Bake for 12 minutes. Set the oven to broil and place the pan on the top rack of the oven. Watch carefully and let the top of the cauliflower brown. Move the pan around and watch carefully so that the pie gets even in color; then broil for about 3 to 4 minutes.

To serve: scoop out one serving of shepherd's pie and top with some avocado slices.

Per serving: 276 calories, 13 g. fat, 28 g. protein, 19 g. carbohydrates

Braised Bison-Stuffed Cabbage Rolls with Sweet-and-Sour Tomato Sauce

Servings: 12

Sweet-and-Sour Tomato Sauce

1 tablespoon grapeseed oil
½ cup finely diced onion
3 cloves garlic, minced
1 tablespoon tomato paste
28-ounce can crushed tomatoes

Salt and pepper
2 tablespoons coconut sugar
½ cup red wine vinegar
2 tablespoons minced basil
1 tablespoon minced parsley

Filling

1 tablespoon grapeseed oil
1 cup finely diced onion
1 cup finely diced zucchini
4 cloves garlic, minced
1 tablespoon tomato paste
Salt and pepper

1½ cups cauliflower, blanched and riced
2 tablespoons parsley
2 pounds ground bison
1 egg
2 green cabbage heads

Preheat oven to 350°F.

MAKE THE TOMATO SAUCE:

Heat a large saucepan to medium-high. Add the grapeseed oil, then add the onion and sauté until translucent. Add the garlic cloves and sauté for 1 minute. Add the tomato paste and stir well to incorporate. Add the crushed tomatoes and stir well. Season with salt and pepper to taste. Cook for about 20 minutes, stirring occasionally. Add the coconut sugar, vinegar, basil, and parsley. Cook for another 5 minutes, take off the heat, and set aside.

MAKE THE FILLING:

Heat a large sauté pan to medium-high. Add the grapeseed oil. Add the onion and zucchini and sauté until they are soft; add the garlic and sauté for 1 minute. Add the tomato paste and stir to combine. Add 1 cup of the sweet-and-sour tomato sauce; cook for another minute or two to meld the ingredients. Season with salt and pepper to taste and set aside.

Put the sautéed vegetables in a large mixing bowl, add the cauliflower rice, parsley, ground bison, egg, and salt and pepper to taste. Mix together and set aside.

Bring a large pot of water to a boil; season it with kosher salt. Remove any damaged outer leaves from the cabbage and set aside. Cut out the core of the cabbage heads and remove the leaves from the head, being careful to keep them intact. Blanch the cabbage leaves in the salted boiling water for about 5 minutes until soft, then rinse them under cold water and pat them dry. Cut out the tough inner stem from each leaf. Line up each leaf on a large cutting board and overlap the bottoms where the stem was removed so that the leaf is intact again.

Scoop out ½ cup of the meat mixture and place into the bottom half of each cabbage leaf. Fold over the side and roll up the bottom part of the leaf; continue to tuck and roll until the meat is completely covered.

Line the bottom of a large baking casserole pan with the large damaged leaves that you set aside. Place the cabbage rolls in the pan snugly next to one another so that the seam side of the roll faces down. Cover with the sweet-and-sour tomato sauce.

Bake for 1 hour.

To serve: divide into 12 equal servings. This should equal about 2 stuffed cabbage rolls per serving, depending on the size of the cabbage.

Per serving: 223 calories, 4 g. fat, 26 g. protein, 14.5 carbohydrates

Roasted Halibut with Tomato, Caper, and Olive Tapenade

Servings: 2

Cooking spray
Two 5-ounce skinless, boneless
  halibut fillets
¼ teaspoon paprika
¼ teaspoon turmeric
¼ teaspoon coriander
Zest of 1 lemon
Salt and pepper

Juice of 1 lemon
1 tablespoon minced cilantro
1 clove garlic, minced
1 finely diced tomato
1 tablespoon chopped capers
2 tablespoons chopped green olives
½ tablespoon olive oil

Preheat oven to 350°F.

Coat a baking sheet with cooking spray and place the halibut fillets on it. Mix the paprika, turmeric, coriander, lemon zest, and salt and pepper to taste, and sprinkle evenly over the fish. Bake for 10 to 12 minutes until medium.

In a medium-sized bowl, mix together the lemon juice, cilantro, garlic, tomato, capers, green olives, olive oil, and salt and pepper to taste. (The capers and olives are salty, so taste before adding salt; you may not need any.) Let sit and marinate about 15 minutes.

To serve: divide the tomato mixture in half and serve each half over 1 piece of fish. The tapenade can be also served with any roasted or grilled vegetable of your choice.

Per serving: 227 calories, 7.4 g. fat, 29.5 g. protein, 2.4 g. carbohydrates

Yuzu Salmon Sashimi

Servings: 2

6 ounces skinless, boneless wild
  salmon, cut into ¼-inch slices
2 tablespoons yuzu juice
Salt and pepper
¼ teaspoon minced jalapeño
  pepper

1 teaspoon olive oil
1 tablespoon minced chives
½ tablespoon toasted sesame seeds

Lay out the salmon slices overlapping slightly on a plate.

Pour the yuzu juice over the fish, followed by a little salt and pepper and the jalapeño. Let sit for 5 minutes.

Top with the olive oil, chives, and sesame seeds.

To serve: eat immediately.

Per serving: 184 calories, 9 g. fat, 17 g. protein, 0 g. carbohydrates

Grilled Chicken Satay with Almond Butter Dipping Sauce

Servings: 12

Chicken Satay

2 tablespoons minced shallots

1 tablespoon minced ginger

3 cloves garlic, minced

1 can coconut milk

Zest and juice of 3 limes

¼ cup soy sauce

1 tablespoon coconut sugar

Salt and pepper

1 pound chicken tenders

Almond Butter Dipping Sauce

1 tablespoon minced shallots

1 teaspoon minced ginger

1 clove garlic, minced

½ can coconut milk

Cooking spray

Zest and juice of 2 limes

3 tablespoons soy sauce

1 tablespoon coconut sugar

½ cup almond butter

Heat oven to 375°F.

PREPARE THE CHICKEN SATAY:

Place the shallots, ginger, garlic, coconut milk, lime zest and juice, soy sauce, coconut sugar, and salt and pepper to taste in a large glass bowl and whisk well. Place the chicken tenders in the marinade and coat. Cover with plastic wrap and let marinate overnight.

MAKE THE DIPPING SAUCE:

Place the shallots, ginger, garlic, coconut milk, lime zest and juice, soy sauce, coconut sugar, and almond butter into a food processor and puree until smooth.

Coat a sheet tray with cooking spray. Remove the chicken tenders from the marinade and wipe off the excess marinade. Lay the tenders on the sheet tray and bake for 7 minutes.

To serve: divide the tenders into 12 servings and enjoy.

Per serving: 172 calories, 12 g. fat, 12 g. protein, 5 g. carbohydrates

Poached Shrimp Salad

Servings: 6

Poaching Liquid

1 pound shrimp, deveined
2 bay leaves
1 teaspoon whole black peppercorns
5 sprigs thyme

1 shallot, peeled and sliced
5 whole garlic cloves, peeled
2 tomatoes, quartered
2 sprigs tarragon

Salad

3 tablespoons minced red onion
½ cup thinly sliced cucumber
½ cup finely diced avocado
1 teaspoon minced garlic
1 tablespoon minced dill

1 tablespoon minced parsley
1 teaspoon minced fresh oregano
1 teaspoon olive oil
¼ cup lemon juice
Salt and pepper

MAKE THE POACHING LIQUID:

Remove the shells from the shrimp. Place the shells in a large saucepan. Set the shrimp aside. Cover them with 4 quarts water. Add the bay leaves, peppercorns, thyme, shallot, garlic, tomatoes, and tarragon. Simmer over low heat for 30 minutes and strain. Reserve the poaching liquid.

MAKE THE SALAD:

Pour the poaching liquid back into the large saucepan and bring to a low simmer. Add the shrimp and cook for about 3 minutes until just done; do not overcook. Remove from the liquid immediately, place on a sheet tray, and place in the refrigerator until completely cool.

Once cooled, cut the shrimp into bite-sized pieces. Toss the onion, cucumber, avocado, garlic, dill, parsley, and oregano. In a small bowl, combine the olive oil, lemon juice, and salt and pepper to taste, then pour over the salad and toss. Let sit for at least 30 minutes to let the flavors come together.

To serve: divide into 6 servings and enjoy.

Per serving: 108 calories, 3.8 g. fat, 15.5 g. protein, 2 g. carbohydrates

Pea and Edamame Hummus

Servings: 10

¾ bag (12 ounces) frozen peas, thawed
¾ bag (12 ounces) frozen edamame, thawed
1 cup chopped avocado
½ cup chopped mint
4 cloves garlic, chopped

Zest and juice of 2 limes
1 tablespoon olive oil
1 tablespoon tamari sauce
1 teaspoon sambal
Salt and pepper
Water as needed

Place the peas, edamame, avocado, mint, garlic, lime zest and juice, olive oil, tamari sauce, sambal, and salt and pepper to taste in a food processor and puree. Gradually add water a couple of tablespoons at a time as needed to allow the ingredients to blend. You want a thick but easily spreadable consistency.

To serve: serve with any fresh vegetables on hand (carrots, broccoli, cauliflower) or eat by itself!

Per serving: 104 calories, 4.7 g. fat, 6 g. protein, 10 g. carbohydrates

Spicy Teriyaki Wild Salmon Jerky

Servings: 4

½ pound boneless, skinless wild salmon

Marinade
¼ cup soy sauce

1 tablespoon coconut sugar

1 teaspoon paprika

Zest of 1 lemon

1 tablespoon rice wine vinegar

2 teaspoon sambal

2 cloves garlic, finely grated

½ teaspoon finely grated ginger

Using a very sharp knife, cut the salmon against the grain into ½-inch-thick slices.

MAKE THE MARINADE:

Place the soy sauce, coconut sugar, paprika, lemon zest, vinegar, sambal, garlic, and ginger into a large glass bowl and whisk well to combine. Place the salmon in the marinade and coat all the pieces. Cover with plastic wrap and marinate overnight.

Preheat oven to 175°F.

Lay paper towels on a sheet tray, remove the salmon slices from the marinade, and place them on the paper towels. Put another layer of paper towels over the fish and pat the salmon dry. Remove salmon and paper towels from sheet tray.

Line the sheet trays with parchment paper and coat them well with cooking spray. Lay the salmon pieces on the parchment paper, leaving about an inch space around each piece.

Cook them in the oven for 90 minutes; then take them out and flip each piece over carefully. Put back in the oven for another 90 minutes.

Remove from the oven and let cool.

To serve: enjoy! The remaining salmon jerky can be stored in an airtight container for up to a week. Make sure the jerky is completely cooled before storing.

Per serving: 115 calories, 4.65 g. fat, 13.25 g. protein, 4 g. carbohydrates

Taco Turkey Lettuce Wraps with Cilantro Lime Sauce

Servings: 6

Cilantro Lime Sauce
½ cup Greek yogurt
¼ cup lime juice

¼ cup minced cilantro
Pinch of salt

Filling
¾ tablespoon olive oil
¼ cup minced onions
1 tablespoon minced jalapeño
  pepper
Salt and pepper
2 cloves minced garlic
2 minced scallions

1 pound ground white meat turkey
1 tablespoon ancho chili powder
¼ teaspoon cumin
½ teaspoon coriander
Pinch cayenne
1 head butter lettuce

MAKE THE CILANTRO LIME SAUCE:

Combine the yogurt, lime juice, cilantro, and salt in a bowl, stir, and set aside.

MAKE THE FILLING:

Heat a small sauté pan over medium heat and add ½ teaspoon of the olive oil. Add the onions and jalapeños, and sauté until they are soft. Season with salt and pepper to taste, add the garlic, and sauté for 1 more minute. Spoon into a large bowl, stir in the scallions, and set aside.

Put the skillet back on the heat and add the remainder of the olive oil. Add the ground turkey and break it apart; season with salt and pepper to taste. Add the chili powder, cumin, coriander, and cayenne. Add the sautéed vegetables and stir to combine.

To serve: cut off the core of the butter lettuce and lay out the lettuce leaves. Spoon 2 ounces of filling into each leaf and 1 tablespoon of cilantro lime sauce on top. Each serving is 2 tacos.

Per serving: 160 calories, 9.6 g. fat, 17 g. protein, 1 g. carbohydrates

part three

THE 25DAYS WORKOUT:
Your "Best You Blueprint"

chapter seven

The Workout Rules You Need to Know

N ow that you know how to get your nutrition on the right track using the 25Days Diet, it's time to bring your exercise up to speed. To make that happen, you'll be doing some form of activity each and every day throughout the twenty-five days. In a nutshell, here's all you need to know.

The 25Days Workout *Simplified*!

The biggest plus to the 25Days Workout is in its effortlessness. If you're expecting some lengthy, convoluted program that changes every week—the same type of routines my brain had to step away from in the past due to memory loss—you're about to be incredibly disappointed. Simply put:

+ For twenty-five days, you'll be alternating between two types of workouts: what I like to call a **Primary Day** workout and a **Secondary Day** workout.

  + When you do a **Primary Day** workout, you'll be performing a routine of five strength-based exercises to build lean muscle and boost your metabolism.

  + When you do a **Secondary Day** workout, you'll be engaging in a shorter routine that focuses more on conditioning and recovery.

That's it. If you have zero interest in what makes the routines in the 25Days Workout unique, I'm not offended. You're eager to get started, and I can respect that. So feel free to move on to the next chapter to find out what type of activities you'll be doing each day. Otherwise . . .

The 25Days Workout *Magnified*!

First things first: Since the 1980s, exercise programs have become so focused down to the point that most people are led to believe there is only one way to accomplish one thing—and that's inaccurate. There is no such thing as the perfect workout. That said, the 25Days Workout isn't *the* workout.

It's *a* workout.

But I'm willing to bet it's a workout that's far superior to the one you're using now.

How can I make that claim? Well, for starters, I think it's fair to say that you're reading this book because you haven't found a solution to reaching your fitness and health goals. But more important, I'm confident of its efficiency because of how well rounded the workout is—and how successful it's been for keeping both me and my clients in top shape.

If you look at most exercise programs—especially the ones you've most likely tried and failed with—many are typically slanted in one specific way. Maybe it's that weight-training class you love, or perhaps you're the type who puts her faith in a spin or yoga class every single day. No matter what the activity, there's a repetitiveness to most: day in and day out, doing the same activity over and over and over again.

The problem is this: I don't care how much you love your spin class or whatever new strength-training workout you're currently trying. I don't even care how effective whatever you swear by to stay in shape might be. It's a simple fact that any single discipline performed a certain way without any breaks or changes—one that never allows you to switch between anaerobic exercise (any intense activity you can do for only up to two minutes) and aerobic exercise (otherwise known as cardio, which uses oxygen as its main energy source and can be performed for a much longer duration)—will burn only one end of the candle instead of both at once.

Most programs never have a yin to their yang. They don't have an opposing voice, if you will, to what they're putting your body through.

Stick with a program that meets that criterion for too long, and you're setting yourself up for developing muscular imbalances, as well as overworking certain muscles and joints to the point where you'll be more susceptible to injury. But it's what you're doing to your mind that matters most to me.

Better Your Body, Better Your Brain!

How many times have you traveled to work—a routine trip you make every day—arrived safe and sound, and then thought to yourself: "I don't remember any of the trip that I took getting here."

If you force yourself to think about it, would you remember every detail of the train ride or drive in? Could you recall everything that you saw along the way? Probably not. In fact, I'll wager you don't remember anything. It's the type of realization that makes you ask yourself: "How did I mindlessly get here in the first place?"

The reason is this: we become such a hamster on a wheel that our brains begin to knock out all of the outside influences around us. It's what keeps you from seeing all of the signs along the road. It's what prevents you from remembering every detail about your journey. It's a zoning-out process that comes in handy for maintaining your sanity during the mundane, repetitive tasks that we do all the time.

Doing the same type of workout over and over again triggers that same hamster-on-a-wheel mind-set. When you don't exercise in a way that engages your brain, it checks out. If that happens, it doesn't just make you more susceptible to using poor form, performing an exercise incorrectly, or not pushing yourself as hard as possible, robbing you of maximum results; it also opens the door for possible serious injury by keeping you from being aware of your areas of weakness.

See, no matter if you're new to exercise or an advanced exerciser, everyone has some form of imbalance in his or her body. For instance, my imbalance is too little flexibility. It's something that I've always known I have to work on more and more, and something I always need to stay aware of when exercising so I know my limits and always make room for stretches that can help me become more pliable.

When you mindlessly go to the same type of workout day in and day out, and the only thing you're focused on is making it through a class, or running or cycling a certain distance, or lifting a certain amount of weight, at some point your brain becomes oblivious to all of the outside influences. If it believes there's nothing it needs to focus on but that single criterion, it stays hyperfocused on that one criterion, almost to the point of being involuntary.

It zones out to everything else and leaves you unaware of the other areas of yourself that you need to focus on.

Does that mean you could injure yourself? Not necessarily. But if you're going to hurt yourself, it's more likely to happen when you're in a place of being unaware. In other words, if you don't even realize at the end of your workout how you got there, you're opening the door to a possible injury.

That's just one way the 25Days Workout is unique. Even though you'll be asked to flip-flop each day between just two types of workouts (strength training or a conditioning routine), you'll be performing routines of different lengths and different intensities involving a series of exercises and movements.

By varying your routines each and every day, you'll not only become more well rounded from a fitness standpoint, but also you'll be pulling your brain off the hamster wheel. You'll be creating a new "brain wrinkle" that will keep you engaged and aware, so you get more from each workout and are less likely to hurt yourself. But that's not the only benefit of the routines I'm about to reveal.

The 25Days Workout Edge

It Starts Where *You* Begin

Most exercise programs expect you to do this chunk of training at the beginning that seems almost insurmountable. But 25Days flies in the face of convention by doing something nobody else bothers to try: it lets you exercise appropriately from where your starting point is, instead of fitting you into a particular mold and expecting you to pull off a miracle.

What's different about the routines in 25Days is that even though you'll be asked to do a certain amount of exercises for a specific number of repetitions and sets, it doesn't matter to me if completing the workout takes you an entire hour or just ten minutes—it's entirely up to you.

You are free to go at whatever pace you need to go at, so long as you always finish what is asked of you to do for the day. It's that perk that allows you to start at a pace—from the very first day you initiate the program—that's entirely comfortable for you.

It's What I Call "Celebrity-Proven" Convenient

One of the greatest strengths of the 25Days Workout is that it can virtually be performed anywhere, making it completely excuse-proof. That's because all the exercises require nothing more than your body weight as resistance, a stretch cord, and just a few ordinary items you can find anywhere you go.

Each of the routines is tailor-made to be as user-friendly and easily accessible as possible, while also being incredibly efficient because, well, they have to be! Most of my clients are usually in places such as movie sets or backstage at concerts, where access to gym equipment simply isn't on the menu. In fact, my high-profile clients have performed my 25Days Workout routines practically everywhere *but* inside a gym, from parking lots, concert arenas, and tour buses to trailers, TV and movie sets, and hotel rooms. I've even had a few workouts that took place in a hotel lobby.

The workout is designed so that all I need is an empty space, because it's my job to make sure that my celebrity clientele can get in their workouts when it fits their schedules and locations for the day. Because of that convenience, if my workouts are able to keep my celebrity clientele in performance shape while they maintain a schedule of eighteen-hour days, seven days a week, just imagine what they'll do for you.

IT'S A BRAIN BOOSTER

Research has shown that resistance training can keep your brain sharp by having a significant effect on transitions in both selective attention and conflict resolution, particularly in older women.[*] Also, a single bout of moderate-intensity exercise for as little as thirty minutes has been shown to shorten the time needed to complete a test[†] by improving certain aspects of cognition (most prominently memory), reasoning, and planning.

How does this happen? Simple: as you train your muscles, you're also working your brain and spinal cord, otherwise known as your central nervous system. By performing more complex and intense exercises or routines (which is exactly what you'll find in 25Days), you place a greater amount of stress on your CNS, which adapts as a result.

That adaptation leads to a variety of cranial changes, including more motor unit recruitment, greater neural stimulation, and an improved level of communication between your receptors (specialized cells at the ends of nerve fibers that detect change) and effectors (any part of your body that has to respond to those changes). In a nutshell, when a receptor gets stimulated, it shoots a signal through your nerve cells to report

[*]N. Fallah et al., "A Multistate Model of Cognitive Dynamics in Relation to Resistance Training: The Contribution of Baseline Function," *Annals of Epidemiology* 23, no. 8 (2013): 463–68, doi:10.1016/j.annepidem.2013.05.008, Epub July 3, 2013.
[†]Bijli Nanda, Jagruti Balde, and S. Manjunatha, "The Acute Effects of a Single Bout of Moderate-Intensity Aerobic Exercise on Cognitive Functions in Healthy Adult Males," *Journal of Clinical and Diagnostic Research* 7, no. 9 (2013): 1883–85, doi:10.7860/JCDR/2013/5855.3341, Epub September 10, 2013.

to your brain, which then tells your body how to respond. By properly training your CNS on a regular basis (which you'll be doing every other day in this program), you're helping your brain communicate more efficiently with your body.

It's a Head-to-Toe Turnover

When you look at the best athletes in the world, the best sprinters and long-distance runners lift weights, and the strongest weight lifters stretch and do some form of cardio. That's because elite athletes understand that greater ranges of motion and body awareness help to promote what they're doing, no matter what that sport or activity is. They realize the importance behind varying the styles and kinds of workouts they're doing.

They recognize that to succeed, it's not just about breaking a sweat; it's about giving the body time to heal. It's about incorporating the right movements that allow it to be flexible and agile. It's about throwing in techniques that teach the body better coordination and improve its balance. And last but never least, it's about putting in the necessary work to make the body explosive and strong.

The best program is one that accounts for all those things; one that divides your time the right way so that you're able to improve all of those necessary areas all at once. One that involves all of the above to get both your body and your brain engaged. Combined, the routines that make up the 25Days Workout do exactly that.

It Makes Your Muscles Get Along—So They Get Strong

A lot of workout programs are filled with exercises that isolate individual muscle groups, such as the biceps or triceps. That's not the case with the strength-training routines in the 25Days Workout, which rely on more multijoint movements; exercises that work several muscle groups at once.

Don't get me wrong: these type of isolation, single-joint moves have their place, if, say, you're a bodybuilder who needs to put the finishing touches on a specific muscle group or someone with a muscular imbalance who needs to bring a weaker muscle group up to speed. But if that's not you, then using a program packed with isolation exercises can be a waste of your time.

Using multijoint movements like the ones in 25Days makes it far easier to train your entire body in less time using fewer exercises. They also prepare your body for more real-life situations where your muscles need to work together to perform a particular task. After all, when was the last time you needed to curl something up to your shoulder? That's right: never.

It Burns More Calories, Even When You're off the Clock

Another key reason that 25Days relies on multijoint exercises is that they're more efficient at waking up the central nervous system, as well as making sure you burn calories every single hour throughout the entire twenty-five-day program. See, it takes energy to move, but, contrary to what many people believe, your body doesn't instantly derive energy directly from the foods you eat. Instead, it receives energy mostly in the form of adenosine triphosphate (ATP), an immediate form of chemical energy, used for all cellular function, that's synthesized from foods. ATP is what's behind making your muscles contract, so that when you start any workout, your body relies on ATP to keep you going.

The problem is: your body can store only a tiny amount of ATP in your muscles. So when you begin exercising, it uses up that amount up within just six to ten seconds. If, after ten seconds, you stop to rest, your body uses an energy pathway known as the ATP-CP system, which resynthesizes ATP using a finite amount of creatine phosphate, a high-energy compound also stored in your muscles relied on only during short, high-intensity activity. But if you're planning on working out for longer than ten-second spurts, your body has no choice but to turn to two other energy pathways to continue resynthesizing the ATP needed to fuel your workouts:

The Anaerobic Energy Pathway (or Glycolysis). When you perform any high-intensity exercise, it reduces the amount of oxygen-rich blood to your muscles. Fortunately, the anaerobic energy pathway doesn't require oxygen and creates ATP purely from glucose, or stored carbohydrates. It's able to produce ATP quickly and rapidly for short, high-intensity bursts of activity lasting thirty seconds to roughly three minutes, max. After that, the lactic acid that's produced as a by-product of the process builds up within the muscles and generates muscle pain and fatigue, making it extremely hard to maintain the intensity.

The Aerobic Energy Pathway (or Aerobic Metabolism). When you perform any type of less intense (or long-duration) exercise or activity, ATP gets produced primarily by the aerobic pathway, which uses oxygen to convert mostly carbohydrates and fat into ATP. Because this pathway uses your circulatory system to get oxygen to your muscles before it creates ATP, it runs much more slowly than the anaerobic energy pathway. But as long as your body has access to oxygen and enough carbs and fats to use for fuel, it lets you perform aerobic activities for a longer period of time.

You actually use a combination of all three of these systems during physical activity, depending on the duration and the intensity of what you're doing. But many people make the mistake of sticking with activities that rely more on the aerobic energy pathway because they believe it's the best route to weight loss. So they trudge along for hours on a treadmill, bike, or stepper at a low-intensity, steady rate. What they fail to recognize is that doing high-intensity, strength-training exercises that rely on glycolysis for energy may burn fewer calories during your workout, but they force you to burn a lot more afterward.*

It works like this: EPOC (otherwise known as excess postexercise oxygen consumption) is the amount of oxygen it takes to restore your body

*Christopher B. Scott, "Quantifying the Immediate Recovery Energy Expenditure of Resistance Training," *Journal of Strength and Conditioning Research* 25, no. 4 (2011): 1159–63, doi:10.1519/JSC.0b013e3181d64eb5.

to a normal state of homeostasis—the state of balance your body constantly maintains—after intense exercise. Even though you might need a rest after performing the right type of high-intensity routine, your brain never stops. Behind the scenes, it's hard at work telling your body to do everything from rebalancing the oxygen levels in your blood and rebuilding damaged tissues to resynthesizing glycogen to be delivered to the muscles and producing ATP.

All that extra effort takes a lot of energy that causes you to burn significantly more calories throughout the twenty-four to forty-eight hours after your workout. Using the multijoint strength-training exercises in 25Days (and the high-intensity way you'll be asked to perform them), you'll place a greater demand on your body's anaerobic energy pathways,* which in turn will raise your body's need for oxygen after you're through. In fact, by boosting the EPOC effect, you can expect to burn an additional 10 to 15 percent of calories after the hard work you already completed.

It Keeps Your Heart in High Gear

You might say I'm partial when it comes to paying attention to how hard my heart is working during exercise because of what I've been through, but it's more about getting clients the best results possible.

One form of strength training I'm fond of is where you arrange exercises in an order that alternates between lower-body and upper-body exercises. This style of training—known as peripheral heart action, or PHA training—makes your heart work harder than usual at pumping blood throughout your body. All that extra effort takes energy, causing your body to burn even more calories while you simultaneously strengthen your heart. It's a two-for-one deal that's hard to beat.

Another benefit of PHA training is that it's equal to high-intensity interval training (HIIT), which has become incredibly trendy over the

---

*J. LaForgia, R. T. Withers, and C. J. Gore, "Effects of Exercise Intensity and Duration on the Excess Post-Exercise Oxygen Consumption," *Journal of Sport Sciences* 24, no. 12 (2006): 1247–64, doi:abs/10.1080/02640410600552064.

last decade. According to a recent study[*] performed by the Department of Biomedical and Neuromotor Sciences at Italy's University of Bologna, PHA whole-body resistance training was found to be just as effective as HIIT at increasing muscular strength and maximum oxygen consumption. In layman's terms: it's just as good at building the lean muscle tissue needed to help raise your metabolism, so you burn fat all day long and boost your VO_2 Max.

Why does that matter? Your VO_2 Max is the maximum amount of oxygen your body can utilize during intense exercise to generate adenosine triphosphate (ATP), the energy source that lets your muscles work continuously as you exercise. Raising your VO_2 Max improves your cardiorespiratory fitness level, which will help you exercise longer, burn more calories during your workout, and leave you feeling less tired afterward as a result.

The 25Days Tweak. The way I've designed both Primary Day workouts, you'll be toning and strengthening either your upper or lower body by using as many different planes, angles, and directions as possible to exhaust your muscles thoroughly. But it's also critical to give your muscles ample time to recover so they can come back stronger and perform harder and faster during your next workout.

That's why what I've done with the 25Days Workout is to *magnify* the PHA approach to exercise.

You see, as much as I love PHA training, if you perform it too often, your muscles never get a chance to heal because you are constantly training your upper and lower body together. And because ultimately I want your muscles to operate at their absolute maximum potential on Primary Days, you need to give them ample time to rest and recover.

The way 25Days is set up, each Primary Day workout focuses on either your upper body or lower body and doesn't repeat itself for ninety-six hours, giving your muscles plenty of time to heal. However, in both

[*]Alessandro Piras et al., "Peripheral Heart Action (PHA) Training as a Valid Substitute to High Intensity Interval Training to Improve Resting Cardiovascular Changes and Autonomic Adaptation," *European Journal of Applied Physiology* 115, no. 4 (2015): 763–73, doi:10.1007/s00421-014-3057-9, Epub November 27, 2014.

workouts, there's an exercise thrown in the middle that works the muscles of the opposite half of your body. What this trick does is give whichever muscles you're focusing on that day just a little bit of a reprieve—even if it's only for thirty seconds or so. But more important, it places your body temporarily into a peripheral heart action zone, so your heart works harder and your body burns more calories.

It's Completely Expendable

Wait a minute—did I just say that?

That's right: I'm admitting that you don't have to do the workouts in this book, but you have to do something comparable.

Ready for a little honesty? The truth is, as much as I love the workouts in this book and have witnessed how well they work for my clients, what makes 25Days ideal is that you have far more flexibility to try other workouts—or stick with the programs you're currently using—if that's what keeps you motivated.

I'd never want you to have to tell your friends you can't meet them for a spin or aerobics class, or force you to stop lifting weights or using machines, just because you're following 25Days. In other words, I don't want you to stop doing some of the things you love doing. The great news is, you won't have to; you just need to understand how to substitute the workouts in this book for the routines and classes you may already enjoy, which I'll show you later on.

However, if you're lacking something to do, or ever under the gun for time and don't have another solution, just know that the 25Days Workout is the same ultimate time-saving, problem-solving, full-body workout that gets my clients into star shape.

chapter eight

The Workout Put-Ins/the Cut-Outs

There's a method to the exercise routines within the 25Days Workout. As I mentioned in chapter 7, you'll be alternating between two types of workout days: Primary and Secondary. But before I show you the exercises themselves, it's important to have a better understanding of what you can expect to find within each, as well as get dialed in to a few tricks that will help you achieve even better results.

The 25Days Workout *Simplified*!

✦ On odd days (1, 3, 5, 7, 9, and so on), you'll do a **Primary Day** workout.

✦ On even days (2, 4, 6, 8, 10, and so on), you'll do a **Secondary Day** workout.

On Primary Days

You'll start by doing a ***dynamic warm-up*** consisting of four exercises. You'll run through all four moves—one after the other—twice (with no rest in between) to prepare your body for the main workout.

Next, you'll perform a ***strength-training workout*** consisting of five multijoint exercises done one after the other. At the end, you'll either skip or run in place for thirty seconds and then repeat the five-move circuit for as many times as instructed: three times for beginners, four times for intermediate exercisers, and five times if you consider yourself an advanced exerciser.

This is the only part of the workout you'll be graded on. You'll grade yourself strictly on how much of the strength-training workout you're able to complete each day—and nothing else. You won't be judged on how much or how little you can lift or how long it takes you to complete the workout.

There are two different strength-training workouts: Primary Day A focuses mainly on your lower body, and Primary Day B targets mostly your upper body.

Finally, to ease your body back down, you'll perform a **Crunch-less Core-Down** that consists of three exercises that collectively target your core muscles.

On Secondary Days

You'll perform one of three different types of conditioning workouts, depending on the day:

- ✦ A circuit of six exercises that challenge your cardio.

- ✦ A shorter circuit of three exercises that also challenge your cardio.

- ✦ A low-intensity activity for at least thirty minutes, in addition to a series of stretches I call **Moving Meditation**. These six simple moves will keep your major muscle groups limber, so that you don't experience the muscle tightness that can limit overall results.

For the Best Results. Perform each workout at the same time each and every day, no matter what the workout. If possible, do each and every workout first thing in the morning before eating breakfast. If that's impossible, then choose a time where you have the most energy—and stick to it.

Don't skip a single step of any workout, even if you feel certain portions may not be necessary or you're pressed for time. Trust me when I say that it's all in there for a very important reason.

Make your workout your top focus for the day, over any and all other activities. If you choose to do anything active in addition to your workouts, make sure whatever you're doing isn't so tiring that it affects your workout the next day.

You're done! The next chapter will walk you effortlessly through each exercise and daily routine every step of the way, so I'll see you there. But if you're curious about the components of each workout, why I insist you do every one of them, and the reasons I'm so particular about how and when you exercise, then press on.

The 25Days Workout *Magnified*!

THE PUT-INS

Whether you're doing a Primary Day or Secondary Day workout, both routines break down in their own way for their own reasons. If you're ever in doubt about any portion of the 25Days routines, here's why every piece of the 25Days puzzle matters:

ON PRIMARY DAYS

1. The Dynamic Warm-up

Before you exercise, it's important to prestretch and prepare your muscles with movements that get your blood moving to help prevent injury, minimize muscle stiffness, and improve your overall coordination for what's ahead. That's why it is key to do some form of dynamic warm-up: a series of simple exercises that activate your nervous system, increase your range of motion, and raise your body temperature.

Each of the two strength-training routines within the 25Days Workout begins with a circuit of four movements that do just that, preparing your neuromuscular, cardiovascular, and muscular systems for activity. All it takes is three to five minutes, and your body is primed for peak performance. But more important is the effect the right dynamic warm-up will have on your brain.

When done properly, a dynamic warm-up helps to get your neural patterns firing to recruit muscles in a safe environment before you challenge them using a high-intensity workout. It flips the switch between your mind and your muscles, reminding them how to work together. That way, when you jump into the main strength-training workout portion of 25Days, your brain and body will be more in sync with each other, reducing your risk of injury and raising your overall results.

IF you're thinking about skipping the dynamic warm-up . . .

THEN, well, prepare for fewer results.

First off, it's not just about warming up your body and getting blood into your muscles or making your muscles more pliable—it's about making sure you get the most out of every workout.

Yes, the main benefit of your Primary Day Workouts comes from the five strength-building exercises in the middle. In fact, that's the reason I want you to grade this portion, because it's where you need to perform at your best. However, if you're not doing the dynamic warm-up (or are putting less effort into it than you should be), you'll be preventing your heart from being able to work at its highest capacity during your workout.

If you choose to blow it off or phone it in, I can't stop you. But I can guarantee that if I placed you side by side with somebody who did the dynamic warm-up first, he would not only burn more calories than you but also move faster than you, become stronger than you, and, most important, progress faster than you because his heart is already in that work zone.

2. The Strength-Training Workout

To you, it may just look like five exercises performed one after the other to save time—and you will. But the high-intensity exercises chosen for both strength-training workouts are also multijoint movements that force several muscle groups to work together at once. The more muscles you can incorporate into one workout, the more calories you'll burn overall and the higher you'll raise your metabolism postworkout.

Relying on movements that teach your muscles how to work with one another will also help you build functional strength. That means you'll not only see a difference in the shape and strength of your muscles as you move through the program, but also you'll experience a drastic improvement in your balance and coordination.

In addition to recruiting as many muscle fibers as possible and making them all play nice, the program uses a consistent amount of big central nervous system (CNS) activating exercises that help to make your CNS more efficient. You see, even though your muscles take all the credit for being strong, what decides your strength is how many muscle fibers you can use at a given moment—and that number is determined by your brain. It's your mind that tells your muscles to contract through nerves within the spinal cord and through motor neurons that carry the order to your muscle fibers. The more motor neurons you can activate when working out, the more muscle fibers you'll contract.

Using a program that trains your CNS simultaneously will also improve your intramuscular coordination. When you don't strength train, motor neurons typically discharge randomly, causing your muscle fibers to contract randomly as well. Through the right training, your motor neurons start to discharge in synchronicity, causing your muscle fibers to contract at the same time and making your muscles even more efficient.

IF *the thought of building lean muscle bothers you . . .*

THEN *you need to get over that!*

_____

First off, building muscle doesn't make you look bulky—having too much body fat does. Second, the more lean muscle you have on your frame, the higher your metabolism has to rev, and the more fat you'll burn all day long without even trying.

The bad news: once you reach thirty years of age, the calendar starts to work against you. That's when your body starts losing roughly a half pound of muscle each year, causing your metabolism to decrease by 3 to 5 percent every decade.

The good news: doing some form of strength training two to three times weekly has been shown to prevent that.

The best news: with 25Days, you'll be performing three to four days of strength training, so you'll not only help preserve what you have but add even more metabolism-boosting lean muscle tissue as well.

3. The Crunch-less Core-Down

Because each strength-training workout is an intense program designed to engage your entire body, your heart will be racing faster than normal, your body temperature will be elevated, and your blood vessels will be dilated afterward. End your workout too abruptly, and you never give your body time to come back down to a normal functioning state. It's the reason why some people immediately feel sick or light-headed after an intense routine. It's also the reason that at the end of every strength-training session, you'll be performing a quick routine of three exercises that strengthen your core muscles: the abdominals, the obliques (or love handles), and those in the lower back.

This magnified—yet effective—form of active cooldown is just enough to gradually bring your respiration, body temperature, and heart rate back to normal. At the same time, you'll be allowing just enough blood to circulate vital healing nutrients and oxygen throughout your body. As a result, you'll also experience less soreness after your workout by gradually pushing lactic acid out of your muscles.

ON SECONDARY DAYS

1. The Dynamic Warm-up

Guess what? As important as a dynamic warm-up may be, *you won't be doing any on Secondary Days*. That's because on these days, the workouts you'll be performing—and the cardio and conditioning-based exercises present within each routine—provide the exact same benefits as a dynamic warm-up. So as you exercise, you'll be simultaneously warming up the muscles you'll be using as you go.

2. The Conditioning Workout

Because the high-intensity strength-training routines you'll be doing on Primary Days shock your central nervous system, are more taxing on your joints, and leave your muscles tired and sore, you need to bring your body back into balance. That's why you'll be doing some form of conditioning workout every other day, each designed to help promote a state of constant healing throughout your body.

Why not just take every other day off and rest entirely? Because your body recovers better when it's active than when it's sedentary, for a variety of different reasons. Each of the three lower-impact, joint-friendly conditioning workouts you'll be doing on Secondary Days not only helps to regulate your hormone levels and flush lactic acid from your muscles but also drains your lymphatic system, the network of vessels and bean-shaped nodes that carries nutrients to cells and moves cellular waste to your bloodstream so that it can be eliminated through your kidneys, colon, and lungs.

More important, because high-intensity exercise exhausts your central nervous system, it leaves your muscle fibers weaker the next day as well because the neural network responsible for triggering them to fire and contract is fatigued. That can put you at a greater risk of sustaining injury as well as overtraining if you don't give your CNS a chance to recover properly. By cycling back and forth between strength and conditioning workouts every other day, you'll give your CNS just enough restorative time to recover, so you never find yourself too exhausted to stick with the program and will always be ready for the next day's challenge.

3. Moving Meditation

Stretching your muscles after they're good and warmed up can help your body heal even further. Done correctly, the right mix of movements not only will reduce any lingering aches left behind from exercise but also will lower your risk of injury and let you tap even more of your body's full potential.

Those are just a few of the reasons why I've included a quick six-move stretching circuit at certain intervals throughout the 25Days program. Think of the circuit as a way to get in touch with your body as you simultaneously increase your range of motion in a way that will boost every aspect of your overall performance, from raising your strength and endurance to improving your balance, agility, and speed.

IF you're motivated to move even more . . .

THEN feel free to use this six-stretch routine anytime and as often as you like throughout the entire 25Days program. Doing it every day will help promote healing and prevent injury, and I personally use it seven days a week to stay flexible and injury free.

Because of the way I've arranged the 25Days Workout, you'll be busy doing something active every single day. It's designed specifically to keep your body active and your mind and muscles guessing about what's coming next. That's why it's vital that the exercises I'm asking you to do remain your top focus for the day over any and all other activities you may be considering.

But I get it. In today's "more must be better" society, it's easy to think that pushing yourself just a little harder will produce better results. However, try to squeeze too much into the 25Days program—either by doing more than you're ready to handle or by overengaging in additional activities that may never give your body the time it needs to heal—and your good intentions may end up undermining your results. More important, *doing more could hurt your score*, which will impact how large a dopamine response you get at the end of those off-days.

TO CUT OR NOT TO CUT

If you've already done your workout for the day and you're going to take a hike with your friends in the afternoon or go out dancing later that night, that's fine. There really aren't any off-limits activities when following 25Days. Just as long as you understand two things:

- One, if you're piling on more activities because you want to reach your fitness goals faster, there's no need to push yourself. Just as long as you've made each workout a priority for the day first and foremost (and you're staying true to the 25Days Diet), you'll see results much faster than you expect. You need to have complete faith in the system.

- Two, although I want you giving it your absolute all in every workout (when required to do so), I don't want you going as hard in any other extracurricular activities. Do that, and you run the risk of either overexerting yourself in a way that keeps you from exercising the next day or preventing yourself from getting the best possible score by not giving your body enough rest. Either way, both of those issues could keep you from being consistent with the program and making the most of 25Days. That's why I need you to be aware of what your "perceived exertion" is.

Perceive to Achieve!

As you exercise or perform any activity, I want you to rate how hard you're pushing yourself on a scale of 1 to 10—with 1 being "You're barely trying" and 10 being "As hard as you possibly can go." If you're having trouble breaking down exactly what number to choose, try using the following rated perceived exertion (RPE) scale:

RPE 1 to 2 (very easy): a very slow pace that lets you have a conversation with no problem.

RPE 3 to 4 (easy to moderately easy): an easy pace that lets you have a conversation comfortably with some effort.

RPE 5 to 6 (moderate to moderately hard): a quick, brisk pace that lets you talk, but if you had to sing—forget it.

RPE 7 to 8 (difficult to very difficult): a high-intensity pace where conversation is off the table, but you could throw out short phrases if necessary.

RPE 9 to 10 (maximum effort): an extremely high-intensity pace that makes speaking simply impossible.

With all of the workouts within 25Days (with the exception of what you'll be asked to do on Secondary Day 3, which is your active healing day), I'll be asking you to stay between 6 and 8, which will mean you'll be working at about a 65 to 85 percent range of your capabilities. But for anything extra—that hike with a friend, that pickup basketball game with your kids, that night out to go dancing, and so on—I want you to use your best judgment.

To be honest, most people never run the risk of overtraining, which is why I don't often have to get my clients to dial it back. That being said, I've also had one or two type A personalities who love to test their limits, and if that's you, I don't want you falling prey to being overeager and doing anything that might negatively affect what should be your priority for the day. So here's what I recommend if you're starting 25Days for the very first time:

+ **Stick with light, recreational-level activities for the first twenty-five days.**

+ **Time yourself and limit your participation in any activity to twenty to thirty minutes.**

+ **Check your sweat.** Meaning, if you find yourself doing anything to the point where your shirt's wet, you're probably within the 6 to 8 range, so be careful about how much time you spend in that zone.

Don't worry! Because 25Days will get you into better shape as quickly as the first run-through, I don't want you to be afraid to go all out. You can eventually, but let's not test those limits right away.

What matters more is that I don't want you to risk injuring yourself and having to end the program prematurely, stopping your brain from re-wiring itself. I want that neurological pattern to form, so you stick with the program for life. Eventually, after your second or third time through 25Days, once that neurological pattern is set in place, and you've raised your fitness level into the intermediate or advanced zone, then by all means: go for it.

One Final Point About Your Potential

The more you practice calculating your perceived exertion during any activity, the better prepared you'll be to always know your limitations—and when you can really push yourself.

See, your perceived exertion can change almost by the hour. Some of that is due to where your various hormone levels may be at a particular time of day, what your body is currently processing as energy, and so forth. In other words, there may be a lot of moving parts that decide what your perceived exertion is, so you can't always expect it to be the same.

A great example: When was the last time you saw an athlete who always wins get into a championship position and lose? Maybe he did everything right but just didn't "feel it" that day and had no logical explanation for why he couldn't pull it out. In theory, from a physical standpoint, the athlete might have misread his perceived exertion level, and either thought he couldn't push himself further or thought he wasn't pushing himself enough and burned out sooner than he expected.

Perceived exertion gives you the ability to say, "I know I'm pushing myself at around a six to a seven—and I can still have enough to go another half hour." It also lets you know when you have the pedal pressed all the way down to the floor and there's nothing left in your tank. In other words: it lets you measure your own exertion, so you're able to read it in the moment.

As you use 25Days, know that as you get into better shape, your RPE is going to change. Eventually what once felt like a 6 or a 7 will feel like a 4 or a 5. As you improve your fitness, that range will begin to expand, making the level of fitness you'll be able to achieve one day even higher.

Why Timing Is Everything

Sweat at the Same Time—Every Time

Each day, the activity or exercises you'll be doing may change, but what we're doing with 25Days is building a habitual neurological pattern. There needs to be a consistent programming process in place. That's why one essential strategy is to work out at the same time every day. It's what elicits the best growth hormone release—the substance produced by your body to stimulate lean muscle growth. It's what allows for better protein synthesis, so your body heals faster and more thoroughly. It's what helps rewire your brain to make it even easier to find the time and motivation to exercise.

To be honest, you may already do this because there's only a certain time of the day you can carve out for exercise. But if you have options and tend to fit in your workouts wherever you can, it's important to stick with whichever time you choose at the start of 25Days.

Why? It's all about anticipation.

It works like this: Have you ever noticed a need for something at a certain time of day? Maybe it's that cup of coffee first thing in the morning or that desire to have a cookie that always hits you at three forty-five in the afternoon. Those cravings aren't necessarily because you need caffeine or sugar at those exact moments. They could be because your body is used to experiencing a particular chemical reaction at those specific times of the day.

You see, certain activities, such as eating various types of foods, having sex, or just going to bed, can each cause a chemical reaction within your body. If you make those activities routine, then the body eventually heightens in anticipation; it starts to prepare itself for what's to come.

For example, whenever you drink coffee, it temporarily shrinks your cerebral arteries, which causes the blood in your brain to move at a slower pace from one side to the other. Your brain counteracts that process by opening up those arteries in the presence of caffeine. Drink enough coffee at the same time every day, and eventually your brain starts to anticipate that caffeine-induced constriction and opens up your cerebral arteries around the time you usually have your coffee—even if there's no caffeine in your system.

What 25Days lets you do is take advantage of that brain glitch. Typically, as you exercise, your body's internal temperature and level of the stress-response hormone adrenaline begin to rise. Your brain also starts releasing endorphins (which is believed to be five or six times stronger than the powerful painkiller morphine) and triggers a spike in the release of growth hormone.

Exercising at the same time every day—no matter what workout you're doing—puts your body into a positive state where it starts to anticipate each workout and prepares itself accordingly. Essentially, you teach your body, "Every day, I do *this*, so be ready," which helps to enforce the brain change we're trying to create.

IF you can't work out at the same time each day . . .

THEN don't expect your body to be happy about it.

_____

The whole premise of 25Days is to create a neurological pattern that makes continuing the program for life a natural, effortless action. But I'll be honest: to make this a successful program, I want to you to pull every string and cut every corner to forge a new neurological pattern as fast as possible.

If you choose to work out at different times that are all over the map, you'll prevent your body from taking advantage of eventually anticipating your workouts and preparing itself. It also leaves you at the mercy of wherever your hormone and energy levels may fall whenever you finally exercise. You'll be expecting your body to be "up" no matter what time you call on it to be up. That can lead to mixed results that could negatively affect your daily score and how much of a dopamine release you'll receive at the end of each day.

Why Mornings Matter Most

Ideally, I'd prefer that you exercise first thing in the morning because the best results are achieved when you work out before your day begins.

I'll start with the obvious reasons. Right off the bat, you're exercising at a time when your body is operating at a caloric deficit. With nothing in your stomach, there's no food for your body to utilize for energy, leaving your body little choice but burn through more stored body fat (up to possibly 20 percent more) instead. Exercising before the day gets away from you also makes it impossible to skip. If your workout is the first thing you do when you wake up, then it *always* gets done, no matter how quickly the rest of your day flies.

But if you wait until the middle or the end of your day, the odds are also greater that all of the daily stresses and other BS in your life have already checked in. So instead of focusing on your workout, you may find yourself more focused on burning off all the bad that you did on your diet that day, as well as working off whatever stress you might be under. Based on that fact alone, I guarantee that you won't have the same type of workout at seven o'clock at night that you will at seven in the morning.

But why I prefer mornings goes beyond calories, convenience, and distracting crap. You see, all day long, the foods you take in and the activities that you undertake *after* your workout have a significant impact on all the hard work you put in *during* your workout. By exercising first thing—and *then* eating the 25Days Diet—your body is put into a natural healing state for the entire day. Now it not only has plenty of time to recover but also can immediately utilize the healthy foods you'll be feeding it.

Another big reason I insist that clients break a sweat before breakfast is that by getting up early, you capitalize on what's taking place in your body at that time. Research has shown that a variety of certain hormones and other brain chemicals—such as adrenaline and growth hormone—are much higher during the morning hours. Even though you may not be at your most energetic then, your body is often primed hormonally and ready to make the most of your workout.

IF you can't work out in the morning . . .
THEN pick a time when you feel the most energized.

The point is this: if you know beyond a shadow of a doubt that you hate the mornings, I can almost guarantee that you're not going to wake up an hour early—and that's okay. I don't want you to set up any obstacles on the road to success.

Some days you're going to have a burst of energy at the weirdest times. Whether that vitality is merely perceived or real is irrelevant. All that matters is this: perception is nine-tenths reality. So, if for some strange reason, ten o'clock at night is when you can eat nails and bang out exercise better than at any other time of the day, who am I to disagree? If that's the only time for you to get in your exercise, then do it. So long as you pick a time you think is reasonable and you can stick with it—then that time will work just fine.

chapter nine

The 25Days Routines

A1B2A3B1A2B3A1B2A3B1AB3A.

No, that's not a typo; that's the exact order of the five different workout routines you'll be doing for the entire twenty-five days.

It may look confusing, but I promise you, it's incredibly simple once you get started. However, that unique sequence is meant to confuse your brain and body just enough so that both stay equally challenged and engaged as you carve out a new neurological pattern. Not just during your first time through 25Days, but every time you repeat the program afterward.

The 25Days Routine *Simplified*!

- **On Days 1, 5, 9, 13, 17, 21 and 25,** you'll do **Primary Workout A** to strengthen your lower body. Just turn to page 149 to start.

- **On Days 2, 8, 14, and 20,** you'll do **Secondary Workout 1** (found on page 183).

- **On Days 3, 7, 11, 15, 19, and 23,** you'll do **Primary Workout B** to strengthen your upper body (found on page 167).

- **On Days 4, 10, 16, and 22,** you'll do **Secondary Workout 2** (found on page 193).

+ **On Days 6, 12, 18, and 24,** you'll do **Secondary Workout 3** (found on page 195).

How to Grade Yourself

On Primary Days A and B

During every **strength-training workout**, you'll do a round of 5 exercises in a row, one after the other. For every round you complete that day, you'll earn a certain percentage:

+ If you're a **beginner**, you'll do the circuit **3** times total. You'll do **5 to 8 reps** of each exercise. For every round you complete, give yourself **33⅓ percent**.

+ If you're at an **intermediate** level in your fitness, you'll do the circuit **4** times total. You'll do **8 to 12 reps** of each exercise. For every round you complete, give yourself **25 percent.**

+ If you're **advanced**, you'll do the circuit **5** times total. You'll do **12 to 15 reps** of each exercise. For every round you complete, give yourself **20 percent.**

If you do all your rounds, your total grade is 100 percent.

On Secondary Days 1 and 2

During every **conditioning workout,** what you'll do and how you'll score yourself will vary.

On Secondary Day 1, you'll do a circuit of 6 exercises.

On Secondary Day 2, you'll do a shorter circuit of 3 exercises.

You'll do all of the exercises in a row, one after the other. Whether you're a beginner, intermediate, or advanced, you'll do the recommended number of reps (which range from 8 to 20, depending on the exercise). And for every round you complete that day, you'll earn a certain percentage:

- If you're a **beginner**, do the circuit **3** times total. Each round equals **33⅓ percent.**

- If you're at an **intermediate** level in your fitness, do the circuit **4** times total. Each round equals **25 percent**.

- If you're **advanced**, do the circuit **5** times total. Each round equals **20 percent.**

If you do all your rounds, your total grade is 100 percent.

On Secondary Day 3

Scoring yourself on this day is an all-or-nothing endeavor. You'll be asked to engage in a minimum of 30 minutes of low-intensity activity, followed by a 6-move stretching routine.

If you do both, your total grade is 100 percent for the day. Do only one—or neither—and you earn nothing.

Why so harsh? Because this is the day that some people take advantage of. I've had clients believe that since this is the easiest routine in the workout, it's okay to skip it. But to create a new neurological pattern that will help you stick to a healthy lifestyle in the future, it's imperative that you keep your body primed for activity each and every day. Allowing yourself to rest completely also prevents your body from actively healing, so I don't want you to take this day lightly.

The Ground Rules

Do All of the Required Repetitions for Each Exercise Before Moving On to the Next Exercise, Even If You Have to Stop Briefly and Rest. It doesn't matter if it takes you an entire hour and a half to complete the workout—that's entirely up to you. I'll be honest, though: I don't think it's the best use of your time, but you're free to go at whatever pace you need to go. All I care about is that you complete each workout every day, no matter how long that takes.

25DAYS

145

That said, if you can't complete all of your reps, pause, stand there for a minute to take a breather, and then get right back to it. Do as many reps as you can, and if you have to take another breather, do it. I'm not worried, because your body will eventually acclimate to this workout—so long as you stick with it.

Keep Yourself in the Right Zone. No matter how long your workouts end up taking you, I still need you to push yourself at a pace that keeps your heart rate elevated the entire time. The sweet spot is 65 to 85 percent of your maximum heart rate, or MHR. How do you figure out what your MHR is? Just subtract your age from 220. For example, if you're thirty-five, then your MHR would be 185 (220 – 35 = 185).

Figuring out that number is a whole lot easier with a heart rate monitor—and I should know. As a heart patient, I'm almost never not connected to one. In fact, I've got an onboard computer built into my defibrillator, so I have a heart rate monitor going at all times. But if you're not ready to invest in one, just use the rated perceived exertion (RPE) scale mentioned in chapter 8. If you're exercising at a pace that feels between a 6, 7, or 8 (with 1 being no effort at all and 10 denoting all out), then you're working at about 65 to 85 percent of your capabilities, which is right where you want to be.

Time Yourself as You Strength Train. Even though I just said I don't care how long it takes you to complete your workouts, I still want you to time how long it takes you to complete your strength-training workouts from start to finish and keep track of them. Write down that time on your grade sheets.

Why do I want you to keep track of your time? Ideally, you should always be pushing yourself as hard as possible. Having that number can be an incentive the next time you return to that workout. It's also another great way to help you gauge how far you've come as you move through the program.

Just know this: *I don't want you to always feel you have to always beat your last time.* It's 100 percent if you complete the workout—simple as that. So if you perform each strength-training workout in the exact same time you did it the last time, that's perfectly fine.

Don't Be Afraid to Customize Each Exercise. It's natural to be stronger in one exercise and weaker in another. That's why I've included options for each exercise that can make it either easier or more difficult. So if you feel like you can do more reps of a particular exercise, try a more advanced version of that exercise that may help bring the amount of reps you can do within the range suggested. If you can't seem to pull off the required number of reps of a particular exercise, try an easier version of the move.

IF *you've been feeling light-headed or experiencing low energy during your workouts . . .*

THEN *you're allowed to eat some form of starchy carbohydrates once per day. (I would suggest about a half cup of oatmeal.) However, it has to be around the meal or snack* **prior** *to your workout.*

IF *you feel energized during your workouts but feel completely exhausted coming out of them . . .*

THEN *you're also allowed to eat some form of starchy carbohydrates once per day. However, it has to be immediately after your workout. I would suggest either a plain or apple cinnamon rice cake and a scoop of whey isolate protein powder. Why whey? It's a fast-absorbing protein, so your body can put it to use immediately, unlike most protein sources, which can take hours to absorb.*

What Level Should You Choose?

I could give you the same cookie-cutter advice many programs do and say that if you have less than six months' experience working out, start the 25Days Workout as a beginner. If you have six months to one to two years under your belt, start with the intermediate version and see how it feels.

Finally, if you've been exercising for more than two years, you might be ready for the advanced.

But I'm not going to do that.

Why? Because how far you've come in your workouts previous to using 25Days depends on how hard you were pushing yourself before you arrived here. I've had fit clients with less than six months' experience who needed an advanced program to see results. I've also had clients who had been phoning in their workouts for a decade and had never progressed their fitness beyond beginner level before meeting me.

That said, if you're not sure where you fall, I want you to start the workout using the exercises shown, aim to complete the circuit five times, and see how it feels to you. Your body will tell you pretty quickly if some of the exercises you're doing are too difficult and need to be changed for easier versions, or if you're not quite ready to go the distance of finishing five rounds.

But I don't want you starting 25Days discouraged if you shoot for five rounds, manage to do only three at 20 percent each, and then feel you have to give yourself a grade of 60 percent because you didn't complete two out of the five rounds. Instead, if you finish just three rounds, I want you to accept that you're ready only for the beginner level right now and give yourself 33⅓ percent for each round. Likewise, if you finish only four rounds, that means you're an intermediate exerciser, so stay at that level and give yourself 25 percent for each round.

THE BACK-END BOOST

At the end of the strength-training and conditioning circuits, you'll notice that I'll have you doing either 30 seconds of jumping rope (or mimicking the motion) or Toe Taps: a drill where you run in place and quickly tap your toes in front of you.

Don't skip this part—and treat it with the same importance as every exercise in the circuit. I do this with my own training and with my clients for several critical reasons.

After you finish any circuit of exercises—and you're working hard and pushing yourself—trying to immediately pop back in for another round without giving your muscles a little bit of time to rest can take its toll. If a client isn't very strong to start, I'll notice that by not taking this quick active break, he or she starts moving at a much slower pace and tends to struggle more with certain exercises.

But what I've seen in myself and experienced with my clients is that as you get more endorphins flowing and break a better sweat, you start feeling better during your workout. So by adding this 30-second burst of cardio (just something fast that keeps your pulse elevated and doesn't tire out your muscles), it's restorative and tends to motivate you to run through your next circuit at a quicker pace.

It's a reset moment that reminds your brain of the pace you should be exercising in order to get the best results.

It also guarantees that you won't rest too long between rounds. What I've witnessed with other types of programs that allow people to rest in between circuits is that 30 seconds turns into 60 seconds or 90 seconds. By using 30 seconds of activity as your break between rounds, jumping rope or jogging in place, you'll be less likely to stretch out your rest times.

Primary Day A

DAYS 1, 5, 9, 13, 17, 21, AND 25

DYNAMIC WARM-UP

Run through each of the 4 exercises in order for the required number of repetitions. After you've finished all 4, repeat the circuit again without resting in between for a total of 2 rounds.

1. JUMPING JACKS (50 repetitions total)

2. SKY SHOULDERS KNEES AND TOES (10 repetitions)

3. **BUTT KICK RUNS** (10 total repetitions, 5 each leg)

4. **WIDE STANCE TRUNK TWISTS** (20 total repetitions, 10 to each side)

STRENGTH WORKOUT

LOWER BODY SPECIFIC

Start a timer, and then run through all 5 exercises in order for the required number of repetitions: **beginner, 5 to 8 reps per exercise; intermediate, 8 to 12 reps; advanced, 12 to 15 reps.** After you've completed all 5, jump rope for 30 seconds—that's 1 round!

Repeat for the required number of rounds: **beginner, 3 rounds; intermediate, 4 rounds; advanced, 5 rounds.** After you finish your last round, stop the timer and record your time.

1. **SPARTAN LUNGES**

2. **ROCKING HORSES**

3. **PLANK-UPS**

4. **SPLIT JUMP SQUATS**

5. **MODIFIED FIRE HYDRANTS**

Jump rope for 30 seconds.

CRUNCH-LESS CORE-DOWN

Do each of the 3 exercises in order. Repeat for the required number of rounds: **beginner, 3 rounds; intermediate, 4 rounds; advanced, 5 rounds.**

1. **ALTERNATING SUPERMANS** (20 total, 10 to each side)

2. **SIDE PLANKS** (20 total, 10 to each side)

3. **BIG BICYCLES** (20 total, 10 each leg)

1. JUMPING JACKS

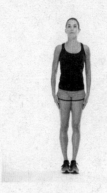

✦ **Start position:** Stand straight with your feet and legs together and arms hanging down at your sides.

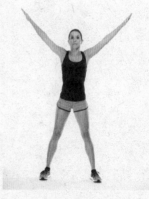

✦ **How to do it:** Swing your arms out from your sides and up above your head as you simultaneously jump up and spread your feet wider than shoulder width apart. Once you land, immediately reverse the motion by hopping back into the start position. That equals 1 repetition.

2. SKY SHOULDERS KNEES AND TOES

+ **Start position:** Stand straight with your feet and legs together and arms hanging down at your sides.

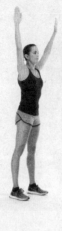

+ **How to do it:** Quickly raise both arms and extend them over your head.

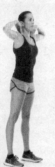

+ Immediately bring down your hands to touch your shoulders,

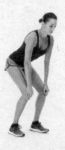

+ and then reach down to touch your knees.

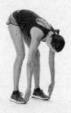

+ Finally, your toes. That's 1 repetition. Return to the start position and repeat the sequence.

3. BUTT KICK RUNS

✦ **Start position:** Stand straight with your legs together and your arms hanging down at your sides.

✦ **How to do it:** Start by running in place.

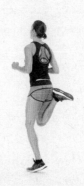

✦ As you bend your legs, pull your heels back and up toward your butt as close as possible. If you can get your heel to hit your butt, that's great. If you can't, just get your heels as close as possible.

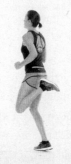

4. WIDE STANCE TRUNK TWISTS

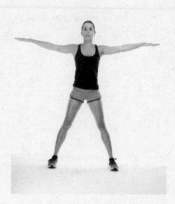

✦ **Start position:** Stand with your legs wide apart with your arms extended straight out from your sides.

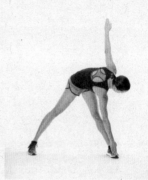

✦ **How to do it:** Keeping your arms and legs straight, twist to your left as you reach down to touch your right hand to your left foot.

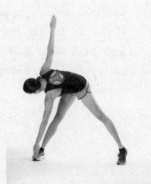

✦ Straighten back up as you simultaneously twist to the right side to repeat the move, this time by touching your left hand to your right foot. (If you can't touch, try to get as close as you possibly can.)

1. SPARTAN LUNGES

✦ **Start position:** Stand straight with your left hand on your left hip and a light dumbbell in your right hand. Curl up the dumbbell so that it's by your right shoulder, with your palm facing forward,

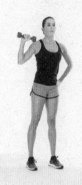

✦ and then press it over your head.

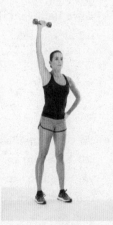

- ✦ **How to do it:** Take a big step backward with your right foot and lower your body

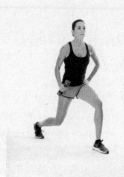

- ✦ until your right knee taps the floor. As you lunge, lower the dumbbell by reversing the press and curl it back down until your right arm is hanging by your side.

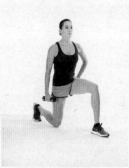

- ✦ Reverse the motion by pressing yourself back into the start position as you simultaneously curl the dumbbell back up to your right shoulder and press it overhead. Repeat the exercise for the required number of repetitions and then switch positions to work the opposite leg.

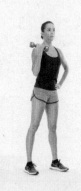

2. ROCKING HORSES

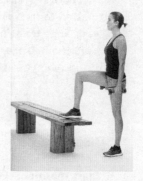

+ **Start position:** Stand in front of a step (or any sturdy object, such as a bench or box) with your feet shoulder width apart and a dumbbell in each hand. Your arms should be hanging down at your sides, palms facing in toward your legs. Place your right foot up onto the center of the step.

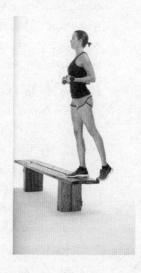

+ **How to do it:** Keeping your right foot flat, push yourself up onto the step, using only your right leg. As you rise, simultaneously curl up the dumbbells to halfway up your chest. At the top, tap your left foot on the step—but don't rest it there. Then reverse the movement by lowering yourself (and the dumbbells) back down into the start position. Repeat for the required number of repetitions and then perform the exercise again, this time by placing your left foot up on the step.

3. PLANK-UPS

+ **Start position:** Get into a classic push-up position, with your hands spaced shoulder width apart and your legs extended straight behind you.

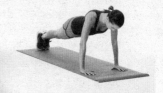

+ **How to do it:** Quickly bend your left elbow and place your left forearm on the floor. Then immediately bend your right elbow and place your right forearm on the floor. (You should

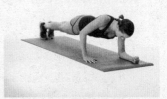

end up in a plank position.) Quickly reverse the exercise in the same order, straightening your left arm first and then your right arm until you're back in the start position. That's 1 repetition.

- Repeat the up-and-down motion, but instead of starting with your left arm, bend your right arm first. Continue alternating from left to right for the duration of the exercise.

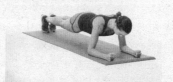

IF the move is too difficult . . .

THEN instead of keeping your legs straight, rest on your knees throughout the entire exercise.

——————————

IF the move is too easy . . .

THEN challenge your stabilization by placing your feet up on either a medicine ball or a Bosu ball. If that's still easy for you, switch positions and place your hands on a medicine ball or a Bosu ball instead.

4. SPLIT JUMP SQUATS

- **Start position:** Stand straight with your feet shoulder width apart and your hands on your hips. Take a small step back with your left foot and a small step forward with your right, so that your feet are about three feet apart.

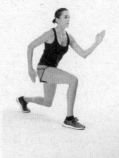

- **How to do it:** Sink into a lunge and then push off with both feet to pop yourself up into the air just high enough to quickly switch the position of your legs. (You should land with your left foot forward and right foot back.)

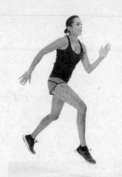

- Sink immediately into a lunge, and push off with both feet to pop up just high enough to quickly bring your legs together.

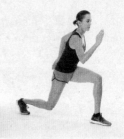

- Land with your feet shoulder width apart, and then, a third and final time, sink immediately into a squat with your arms extended straight in front of you, palms down.

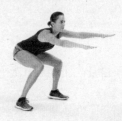

- Stand back up—that's 1 rep—and pause before starting the entire exercise once more.

- **Note:** let your arms swing in the same way they would when running—left leg back, right arm forward, right leg back, left arm forward.

5. MODIFIED FIRE HYDRANTS

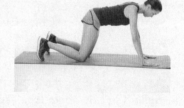

- **Start position:** Get on all fours on a mat or carpeted floor with your hands and knees spaced shoulder width apart. Your hands should be directly below your shoulders, your thighs perpendicular to the floor, and your head staring down directly in line with your spine.

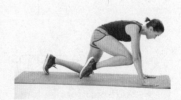

- **How to do it:** Pull your right knee into your chest, and then immediately extend it behind you, keeping your foot raised slightly off the floor. Keeping your right leg as straight as possible, immediately raise it up behind you as high as you can. You should feel a squeeze in the gluteus maximus muscles in your butt and in the hamstring muscles in the backs of your thighs.

25DAYS

161

+ Repeat the move—knee to chest, extending your leg, and then raising your leg as high as possible—until you've completed the required number of repetitions. Then repeat the exercise with your left leg.

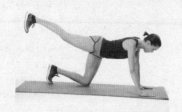

6. JUMP ROPE (30 SECONDS)

+ **Start position:** Hold the rope at both ends, palms facing forward and your arms down at your sides. Stand with your legs together and the middle of the rope lying just behind your heels.

+ **How to do it:** Keeping your arms tucked at your sides, twirl the rope forward, rotating only from your wrists. Once the rope reaches your toes, hop up just enough to allow it to pass underneath—keeping your legs and feet together—and land on the balls of your feet. Repeat the motion at a comfortable pace.

IF you can't jump rope . . .

THEN just mimic the motion without using a rope. Or if that feels awkward, try jogging in place for the same amount of time.

IF skipping for 30 seconds is too easy . . .

THEN don't increase how long you jump, since that will affect your overall time. Instead, try to increase how fast you jump or try doing double jumps, rotating the rope underneath you twice after every hop.

CRUNCH-LESS CORE-DOWN

(THE EXERCISES)

1. ALTERNATING SUPERMANS

✦ **Start position:** Lie flat on your stomach with your arms extended in front of you and your legs straight.

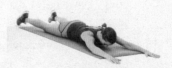

✦ **How to do it:** Slowly raise your left arm and right leg at the same time.

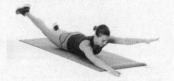

- Hold the position at the top for a moment; slowly lower your arm and leg back to the starting position, and then repeat—this time raising your right arm and left leg. That counts as 1 repetition for each side.

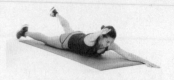

IF you can't master raising one leg and one arm together . . .

THEN try lifting both arms and both legs together. Each time you do, that counts as 1 repetition, so if you choose to do it this way, perform 20 repetitions total.

2. SIDE PLANKS

- **Start position:** Lie on your left side with your legs straight (stacked on top of each other) and your left forearm on the floor to support you. Your left arm should be bent at a 90-degree angle so that your elbow is directly under your left shoulder. Your right hand can either rest along your hip, or you can extend your right arm until it's perpendicular to your torso.

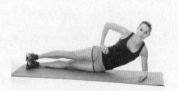

- **How to do it:** Keeping your feet and forearm on the floor, slowly raise your hips until your body forms a straight line from your head through your feet. Pause, and then lower

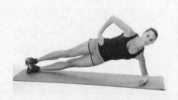

your hips back to the floor. Repeat 10 times and then switch positions to work the opposite side.

IF the move is too difficult . . .

THEN place a ball or a sturdy object about 12 inches high in front of your navel. Then, instead of putting your hand on your hip or extending it above you, place it on top of the object so that you have some support to help you push up. If that's still too challenging, hold yourself in the up position only for as long as you can instead of doing the move for repetitions.

IF the move is too easy . . .

THEN try adding resistance by holding a light dumbbell in the hand that's extended above you, or raise your top leg as well so that you're holding your body in the shape of an X—or try doing both at the same time.

---

3. BIG BICYCLES

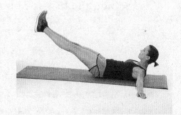

+ **Start position:** Lie flat on your back with your legs straight, arms out from your sides, palms down—you should look like the letter T from above. Raise your head and shoulders off the ground so that you're looking at your feet, and then lift your feet off the floor.

+ **How to do it:** Pull your left knee in toward your chest as close as possible. Then extend your left leg straight up toward the ceiling while keeping your right leg raised.

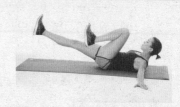

+ Pause, and then, keeping your left leg straight, slowly lower it into the start position (keeping your left foot off the floor) as you simultaneously repeat the move with your right leg, pulling in your right knee, and then extending it straight up

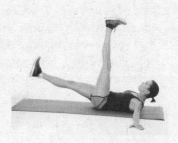

above you. Continue alternating from left to right for the duration of the exercise.

IF the move is too difficult . . .

THEN don't extend your leg toward the ceiling. Just pull each knee up to your chest and then extend your leg back into the start position. If that's still a challenge, try the move with your heels resting on the floor instead of keeping them raised above it for the entire exercise.

IF the move is too easy . . .

THEN try bringing your arms closer in to your body. This tweak will make it harder to stabilize yourself, forcing your core muscles to work harder to keep you balanced as you go. Another way to up the intensity is to try doing the move as slowly as possible. The longer it takes you to lower each leg, the more effort you'll place on your core muscles.

DYNAMIC WARM-UP

Run through each of the 4 exercises in order for the required number of repetitions. After you've finished all 4, repeat the circuit again without resting in between for a total of 2 rounds.

1. **JUMPING JACKS** (50 repetitions)

2. **MOUNTAIN CLIMBERS** (20 total repetitions, 10 each leg)

3. **REVERSE SHOULDER CIRCLES** (20 repetitions)

4. **WIDE STANCE TRUNK TWISTS** (20 total repetitions, 10 to each side)

Strength Workout

UPPER BODY SPECIFIC

Start a timer, and then run through all 5 exercises in order for the required number of repetitions: **beginner, 5 to 8 reps per exercise; intermediate, 8 to 12 reps; advanced, 12 to 15 reps.** After you've completed all 5, jump rope for 30 seconds—that's 1 round!

Repeat for the required number of rounds: **beginner, 3 rounds; intermediate, 4 rounds; advanced, 5 rounds.** After you finish your last round, stop the timer and record your time.

1. **PUSH-UPS**

2. **STANDING BAND ROWS**

3. **HOP SQUATS**

4. **SEATED DIPS**

5. **UPRIGHT ROW/CURLS**

25DAYS

Jump rope for 30 seconds; then repeat the circuit as many times as required.

CRUNCH-LESS CORE-DOWN

Do each of the 3 exercises in order. Repeat for the required number of rounds: **beginner, 3 rounds; intermediate, 4 rounds; advanced, 5 rounds.**

1. HIP THRUSTER HOLDS (20 repetitions total)

2. RUSSIAN TWISTS (20 repetitions total, 10 each side)

3. PLANKS (hold for 30 to 45 seconds)

DYNAMIC WARM-UP

(THE EXERCISES)

1. JUMPING JACKS
See page 151.

2. MOUNTAIN CLIMBERS

+ **Start position:** Get into a classic push-up position with your hands spaced shoulder width apart and your legs extended straight behind you.

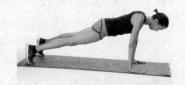

+ **How to do it:** Keeping your hands in place, quickly bring your left knee up toward your chest.

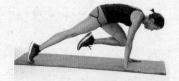

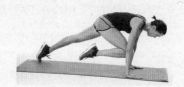

- Then quickly extend it back into the start position as you bring your right knee up toward your chest. Alternate from left to right for the duration of the exercise.

3. REVERSE SHOULDER CIRCLES

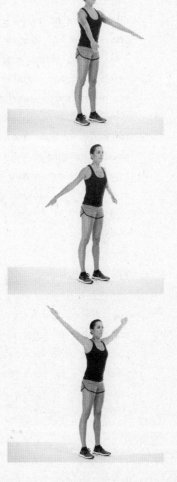

- **Start position:** Stand with your arms extended straight out in front of you, elbows locked and palms facing down.

- **How to do it:** Without bending your arms, rotate them counterclockwise.

- Just imagine that the goal is to have your fingertips trace circles in the air.

4. WIDE STANCE TRUNK TWISTS

See page 154.

STRENGTH-TRAINING WORKOUT

(THE EXERCISES)

1. PUSH-UPS

+ **Start position:** Place your hands flat on the floor, shoulder width apart, keeping your arms straight, elbows unlocked. Straighten your legs behind you, feet together, and rise onto your toes so that the top of the balls of your feet are touching the floor. Your body should be one straight line from your head to your heels, with your eyes looking at the floor.

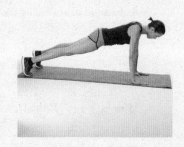

+ **How to do it:** Keeping your arms close to your sides, bend your elbows and lower yourself until your upper arms are parallel to the floor. Straighten your arms to push yourself back up into the start position.

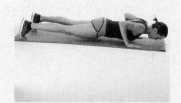

IF the move is too difficult . . .

THEN don't drop to your knees. I don't like modified push-ups from the knees—sometimes called "girl push-ups"—because they aren't as effective at working your muscles. Instead, get into the start position and then touch your left shoulder with your right hand. Get back into position and then touch your right shoulder with your left hand. That equals 1 repetition.

———————

Another modification you can make: get into the start position and then *lower* yourself as slowly as possible. This is called a negative repetition. Once you reach the bottom, keep your knees on the floor, and then roll yourself back so that your butt touches your heels. This will make it easier to get back into the start position.

———————

IF the move is too easy . . .

THEN try placing your feet up on either a step or even a medicine ball or Bosu ball. Another version you can try: each time you push yourself back up into the start position, bring one arm forward as if you were going to slap a friend's hand in front of you. If it helps, you can place something in front of you to tap, such as the edge of a couch or the leg of a chair. Alternate between your left and right arms as you go.

2. STANDING BAND ROWS

+ **Start position:** Loop a resistance band around a doorknob, close the door, and then grab an end (or handle) in each hand. Extend your arms straight out in front of you—palms facing each other—and then step far enough back until you feel equal tension from both ends. Finally, place your feet shoulder width apart, keeping your knees slightly bent for balance.

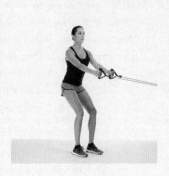

+ **How to do it:** Keeping your back upright, pull your left fist in toward your left side. Don't bend at the waist; the only part of you that should be moving is your arm.

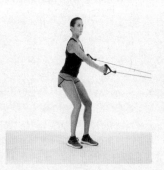

+ Extend your left arm forward into the start position and repeat the move by pulling your right fist in toward your right side. Continue to alternate from left to right for the entire exercise.

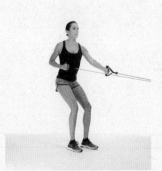

3. HOP SQUATS

✦ **Start position:** Stand with your feet together and your arms down by your sides.

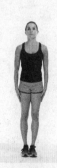

✦ **How to do it:** For this exercise, I want you to think "two hops, drop, and jump." Quickly take two tiny hops up and down on the balls of your feet, keeping your legs together.

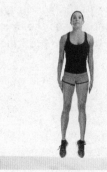

25DAYS

✦ Hop a third time and spread your legs so that you land with your feet slightly wider than shoulder width apart. Immediately squat down as you reach your hands toward the floor (try to touch it if possible), and then jump straight up as high as you can, keeping your arms hanging straight down in front of you. As you descend, bring in your legs so that your feet are together once more when you land. That's 1 repetition.

IF the move is too difficult . . .

THEN don't jump. Once you've gotten down into a squat, just push yourself back up into the start position.

_____

IF the move is too easy . . .

THEN turn the move into a box jump. To start, place a sturdy box or bench in front of you that's between 18 to 24 inches high to start. As you jump up, land directly on the box; then immediately reverse direction and jump off the box back into the start position.

DREW LOGAN

4. SEATED DIPS

◆ **Start position:** Sit on the edge of a bench or sturdy chair and place your hands on the seat on either side of your hips, fingers facing forward. With your feet flat on the floor and your knees bent, slide your butt off the edge until your body weight is supported by your arms.

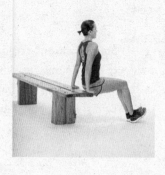

◆ **How to do it:** Bend your elbows and lower your body to the floor, stopping when your arms are bent at a 90-degree angle. Push yourself back up until your arms are straight, elbows just short of locking. That's 1 dip.

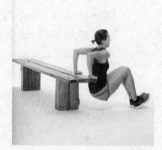

IF *the move is too difficult . . .*

THEN *stop a few inches short of bending your arms 90 degrees and/or try placing your feet a few inches closer to the chair.*

———————————

IF *the move is too easy . . .*

THEN *have a friend place a weight plate or light dumbbell on top of the front of your thighs to add resistance. Another way to intensify the move: instead of keeping your feet on the floor, place your heels up onto another sturdy chair or a stability ball.*

5. UPRIGHT ROW/CURLS

+ **Start position:** Stand holding a pair of dumbbells with your arms hanging down in front of you, palms facing the front of your thighs.

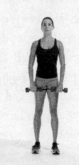

+ **How to do it:** Keeping the dumbbells close to your body, pull up your elbows and raise the dumbbells until they are just below your chin. Imagine that you're making a V with your forearms—elbows high and wrists close together.

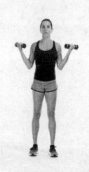

+ Lower the weights back to the start position. Immediately curl up the dumbbells, rotating your wrists outward so that your palms face the front of your shoulders at the top. Curl the dumbbells back down by reversing the motion so that you're back in the start position. That's 1 repetition.

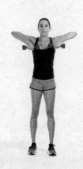

> **IF** the move is too difficult . . .
>
> **THEN** don't curl up the dumbbells. Just raise them up under your chin and lower them—that's 1 repetition.
>
> ---
>
> **IF** the move is too easy . . .
>
> **THEN** instead of curling up the dumbbells, perform what's called a T-fly: raise your arms out to your sides, rotating your wrists outward as you go so that your palms are pointing down toward the floor—you should look like the letter T. Sweep your arms together in front of you so that the ends of the weights touch, return to the T position, and then lower your arms. As they drop, rotate your wrists inward so that you return to the start position (palms facing the front of your thighs).

6. JUMP ROPE

See page 162.

CRUNCH-LESS CORE-DOWN

(THE EXERCISES)

1. HIP THRUSTER HOLDS

+ **Start position:** Lie flat on your back with your legs bent and your feet flat on the floor. Extend your arms out to your sides, palms flat against the floor.

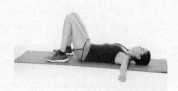

+ **How to do it:** Pressing through your heels, raise your hips off the floor until your body forms a straight line from your knees down through your shoulders. Pause, and then lower back to the floor.

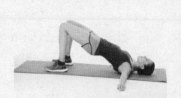

IF the move is too difficult . . .

THEN try skipping the pause at the top of the move and/or come up only a few inches from the floor instead of all the way up.

IF the move is too easy . . .

THEN pause at the top for more than a second. Or try the exercise holding one leg extended straight up above you. After each repetition, switch legs so that the opposite leg is pointing up toward the ceiling and repeat.

2. RUSSIAN TWISTS

+ **Start position:** Sit on the floor with your knees bent and your heels on the floor. Keeping your back flat, slowly lean back until your torso is at a 45-degree angle (From the side, your upper body and thighs should resemble the letter V.) Finally, extend your arms straight out in front of you and clasp your hands together.

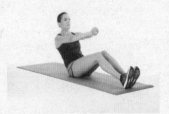

- **How to do it:** Maintaining your balance, slowly twist from the waist and rotate as far to the left as you can comfortably.

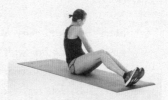

- Slowly rotate back to center and then repeat the move by rotating as far to the right as you can. Keep alternating from side to side throughout the exercise.

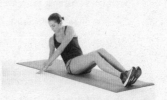

IF the move is too difficult . . .

THEN try placing your feet under a couch or another sturdy object and/or fold your arms over your chest. (The closer in you bring your arms, the less resistance you'll create, which makes the move easier.) If you still find the move hard to do, don't lean back as far.

——————

IF the move is too easy . . .

THEN try raising your feet off the floor an inch and hold them there for the duration of the exercise. Another challenge to try: instead of clasping your hands together, hold a medicine ball instead.

✦ **Start position:** Get into a push-up position with your forearms spaced shoulder width apart and your legs extended straight behind you. Bend your elbows and rest your weight on your forearms—your elbows should be directly below your shoulders. Your body should form a straight line from your head down to your heels.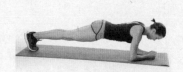

✦ **How to do it:** Keeping your core muscles tight and your neck in line with your spine, hold this position for the required amount of time.

IF the move is either too easy or too difficult . . .

THEN hold the pose for as long as possible without sacrificing your form. If you're a beginner, you should build up to at least 30 seconds, even if it takes a few tries. If you're advanced, aim to hold the pose for at least 1 minute or longer.

DREW LOGAN

IF *you don't want to use either of my Primary Day workouts . . .*

THEN *make sure whatever strength-training workouts you're replacing them with meet the right criteria.*

———————————

First off, if you're thinking about using your own weight-training programs instead of my two strength-training programs, then I'm going to assume you already know how to arrange workouts and understand what a superset is (two exercises performed back to back).

If that's the case, I have no problem letting you use whatever equipment you're currently using for strength training— weights, machines, resistance cords, and so forth—but I need to be clear:

+ **Both Primary Days A and B are arranged in a very specific way that engages your central nervous system.**

+ **Primary Day A is a lower-body intensive routine that focuses mainly on your glutes, calf muscles, hamstrings, and the quadriceps muscles located in the front of the thighs.**

+ **Primary Day B is an upper-body intensive routine that targets mainly the muscles of your chest, back, shoulders, and arms.**

That means if you want to use your own strength-training workout, you'll need to apply the 25Days philosophy to them. So long as you're choosing a series of exercises that hit the same muscle groups, perform them as a circuit, time yourself from start to finish, and put in at least 45 minutes of effort, I'm fine with that. And don't forget to do a dynamic warm-up and cooldown as well.

Ideally, here's what your workout should look like:

+ I'd prefer that you use several pairs of supersets done as a circuit.

- ✦ For Primary Day A, choose a mix of multijoint compound exercises that work your legs evenly. Do no fewer than 2 and no more than 3 supersets.

- ✦ For Primary Day B, choose a mix of multijoint compound exercises that work your upper body, particularly your back, chest, and shoulders. Do no fewer than 3 and no more than 4 supersets.

- ✦ After the first superset, rest 60 seconds or less, and then move to the next superset.

- ✦ Keep your repetitions between 8 and 15, no more and no less. If you can do more than 15, raise the weight; if you can't do 8 repetitions without sacrificing form and putting yourself at a greater risk of injury, lower the weight.

- ✦ Do your substitute workout at the same time you've been working out each day.

The way to score yourself remains the same:

- ✦ If you're a **beginner**, do the circuit **3** times total. Each round equals **33⅓ percent.**

- ✦ If you're an **intermediate** exerciser, do the circuit **4** times total. Each round equals **25 percent.**

- ✦ If you're **advanced**, do the circuit **5** times total. Each round equals **20 percent.**

SECONDARY DAY 1

Run through all 6 exercises in order to meet the required number of repetitions. After you've completed all 6, perform toe taps for 30 seconds—that's 1 round! Repeat for the required number of rounds: **beginner, 3 rounds; intermediate, 4 rounds; advanced, 5 rounds.**

1. **BURPEES** (8 repetitions)

2. **LATERAL HOPS** (20 repetitions total, 10 each side)

3. **HIGH KNEE SPRINTS** (20 repetitions total, 10 each leg)

4. **ALTERNATING DONKEY KICKS** (10 repetitions total for each leg—5 kicks to the front and 5 kicks to the back—for a total of 20 repetitions)

5. **JUMPING WOOD CHOPS** (10 repetitions)

6. **SINGLE-LEG THRUSTERS** (10 repetitions total, 5 each side)

Toe Taps for 30 seconds.

CONDITIONING WORKOUT

(THE EXERCISES)

1. BURPEES

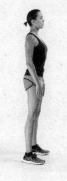

- ◆ **Start position:** Stand with your feet together and your arms down at your sides.

+ **How to do it:** Quickly squat down as low as possible, place your hands on the floor,

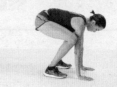

+ and then kick your legs straight back behind you so that you end up in a push-up position. Quickly reverse the motion by pulling your knees in toward your chest, so your feet end up

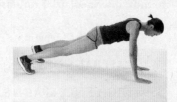

between your hands, and stand up immediately. That's 1 burpee.

IF the move is too difficult . . .

THEN once you've squatted down, try kicking back one leg and then the other (instead of both at once). Another variation that's easier on the back: try standing with your feet wider than shoulder width apart rather than keeping them together.

———

If either of those variations is too hard, just walk your feet back instead of kicking your legs straight back, or walk your hands forward. Either way, you'll end up in a push-up position. Reverse the motion until you're back in a squat position, and then stand up.

———

IF the move is too easy . . .

THEN jump straight up in the air as high as possible—arms extended above your head—instead of just standing back up.

2. LATERAL HOPS

+ **Start position:** Stand with your feet shoulder width apart, knees bent slightly, arms bent at a 90-degree angle.

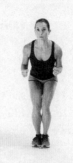

+ **How to do it:** Keeping your legs and feet together, squat down a few inches and then quickly jump to one side.

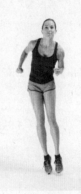

+ As soon as you land, immediately repeat the motion and hop back into the start position. Continue jumping from side to side for the duration of the exercise.

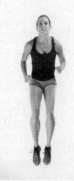

3. HIGH KNEE SPRINTS

+ **Start position:** Stand straight with your feet together and your arms bent at a 90-degree angle.

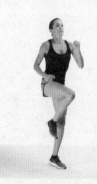

+ **How to do it:** Start running in place.

- As you go, try to bring your knees up to your chest as high as possible while you vigorously pump your arms back and forth like a sprinter.

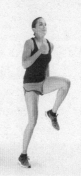

IF the move is too difficult . . .

THEN don't pull your knees up as high, or just run in place as fast as possible without worrying how high your knees rise.

———————————

IF the move is too easy . . .

THEN, as you sprint, do the move with your fingers interlaced behind your head the entire time.

4. ALTERNATING DONKEY KICKS

- **Start position:** Stand with your feet shoulder width apart and your arms bent at 90 degrees.

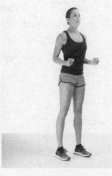

25DAYS

✦ **How to do it:** While balancing on your right leg, pull up your left knee toward your chest and then kick your left leg straight out in front of you.

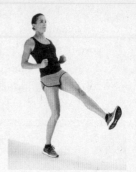

✦ Pull your left knee back in once more, and then kick your left leg straight out behind you. One kick to the front and back equals 1 repetition. Repeat the move with your left leg for the required number of repetitions, and then repeat the exercise with your right leg.

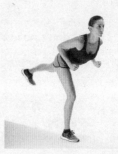

IF *the move is too difficult . . .*

THEN *try holding on to a doorway for support. Other tricks that can make the exercise easier until you master it include not kicking as high or swinging your leg back and forth instead of kicking back and forth.*

———

IF *the move is too easy . . .*

THEN *either try to perform the exercise faster or add repetitions to make it longer.*

5. JUMPING WOOD CHOPS

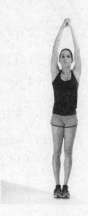

+ **Start position:** Stand with your feet together, arms straight above your head, fingers interlaced.

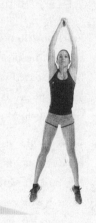

+ **How to do it:** Jump straight up and spread your legs so that when you land, your feet are wider than shoulder width apart.

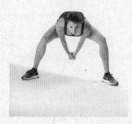

+ As you touch the floor, immediately squat down as you simultaneously swing your arms straight down in front of you. Reverse the motion by jumping up again as you bring together your feet and swing your arms back above your head. Land—that's 1 repetition—and repeat.

6. SINGLE-LEG THRUSTERS

+ **Start position:** Get into a classic push-up position, with your
  hands spaced shoulder width
  apart and your legs extended
  straight behind you.

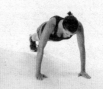

+ **How to do it:** Keeping your
  hands flat on the floor, step your
  left foot forward, placing it as
  close as you can to the outside
  of your left hand; then lower
  your hips briefly.

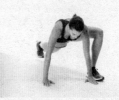

+ Next, step your left foot back
  into the start position, and then
  repeat the move by stepping
  your right foot forward and as
  close to the outside of your right
  hand as possible. Next, lower
  your hips briefly. Continue alternating from left to right for
  the duration of the exercise.

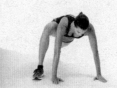

DREW LOGAN

7. TOE TAPS

+ **Start position:** Stand facing a stair (or anything sturdy that's about 4 to 8 inches high) with your feet shoulder width apart, arms down by your sides. Place the ball of your left foot on top of the step.

+ **How to do it:** Think of the move as simply running in place— with a toe tap. Quickly bring your left foot back down to the floor as you spring up with your right foot and tap it onto the step. Reverse the move by quickly bringing your right foot to the floor and tapping your left foot on the step. Continue alternating from left to right as fast as you can go, letting your arms swing naturally back and forth with each step.

25DAYS

IF *you don't want to use my Secondary Day 1 workout . . .*

THEN *make sure that whatever cardio workout you're replacing it with meets the right criteria.*

I really want you to have the power to make choices that fit your lifestyle. So if you want to take a class with a friend or feel like hopping on your bike and seeing how far you can pedal, I'm not going to stop you.

That said, if you want to substitute any high-intensity group class, such as a spin, boxing, or boot-camp-style class, I'm fine with that. But it has to be a high-intensity cardio-specific class that doesn't involve too many strength-training exercises—for example, Pilates or strength-training circuit routines. If you're not into going to a class, any steady-state cardio activity such as running, cycling, lap swimming, or stair climbing will also do. These are the only two rules I have:

1. **Do it at the same time you've been working out each day.**

2. **Whatever activity or class you choose to do *has* to get your heart rate up for a solid 60 minutes.**

I know what you're thinking: "But wait—your workout doesn't take sixty minutes, so why does the activity I'm substituting for it have to be that long?"

Well, that's easy. In terms of calories burned, my workout—and the one you may choose as a substitute—will most likely be equal, even though mine is shorter. Why? For one thing, when most people do any form of steady-state cardio for a long period of time, they typically aren't burning as many calories as they think they are. Also, I have no idea what class you're taking, how good the instructor is, or how effective that class is—so you may be working only some of your muscles as opposed to all of them.

How to Grade Yourself

If you choose to go that route and spend 60 minutes elevating your heart, then completing the class or activity equals 100 percent. If you don't complete the class or activity and stop halfway through, there's no partial time credit.

If the class goes over 60 minutes, you don't receive any extra points—but good on you for sticking it out. However, if the class is under 60 minutes, you need to either fill in the remaining time with an equally high-intensity activity or settle for 0 percent for the day.

SECONDARY DAY 2

DAYS 4, 10, 16, AND 22

Pick any 3 exercises from the list below and create your own 3-move circuit, but include at least 1 exercise with an asterisk. Do each exercise for the required number of repetitions. After you've completed all 3, perform Toe Taps for 30 seconds—that's 1 round! Repeat for the required number of rounds: **beginner, 3 rounds; intermediate, 4 rounds; advanced, 5 rounds.**

*1. **BURPEES** (8 repetitions)

*2. **HIGH KNEE SPRINTS** (20 repetitions total, 10 each leg)

*3. **JUMPING WOOD CHOPS** (10 repetitions)

4. **LATERAL HOPS** (20 repetitions total, 10 each side)

5. **ALTERNATING DONKEY KICKS** (10 repetitions total for each leg—5 kicks to the front and 5 kicks to the back—for a total of 20 repetitions)

6. **SINGLE-LEG THRUSTERS** (10 repetitions total, 5 each side)

Toe Taps for 30 seconds.

Secondary Day 2 is a shorter version of what I'm asking you to do on Secondary Day 1. The repetitions won't change, and you still have to do the same number of rounds, but you have to do only 3 exercises of your choice.

I don't care which moves you choose the first time around—I'll leave the decision up to you—but I recommend that at least one of the moves be a burpee, high knee sprint, or wood chop. These are the hardest exercises of the 6 and the ones that give you the most bang for your buck.

IF you're picking the same three each time . . .

THEN you're robbing yourself of an opportunity.

If I had to bet, you're picking the same exercises to either avoid ones you're not as proficient at or that feel more taxing—or both. If I had to bet, you're probably picking the same exercises and dodging others because you haven't mastered them yet (or maybe they're mastering you!).

That being said, practice makes perfect, and the more you perform these moves, the more proficient you'll become. So don't shy away from the ones you hate—make it a challenge to choose them instead.

IF you don't want to use my Secondary Day 2 workout . . .

THEN know you also have options.

If you don't feel like picking 3 moves and would rather try something else for the day, you can use the same types of cardio-specific options I mentioned on page 192. But instead of finding an activity or class that's 60 minutes long, limit yourself to no more than 45 minutes of activity.

SECONDARY DAY 3

For restorative recovery, perform some form of low-intensity activity—such as flat walking or a light swim—for a minimum of 30 minutes.

Moving Meditation

Do each of the 6 stretches in order as a circuit and hold each stretch for a minimum of 30 seconds—that's 1 round! Repeat for 3 rounds, whether you're a beginner, intermediate, or advanced.

1. **STANDING QUAD STRETCH** (loosens the quadriceps)

2. **MODIFIED FLANK** (stretches the spine)

3. **SINGLE-LEG HAMSTRING STRETCH** (loosens the hamstrings and calves)

4. **HALF LORD OF THE FISH POSE** (stretches the hips, glutes, chest, shoulders, and neck)

5. **COBRA** (stretches the core)

6. **FEET OVER HEAD** (stretches the lower back)

> **IF** you say to yourself, "Wow! I had a great workout!" . . .
> **THEN** you did it all wrong.

Welcome to the easiest of the 5 routines, but don't think it's not as effective as the others. Real growth is achieved during these days of active rest, and its entire purpose is to place your body in a state of active healing. You're not supposed to be challenged on this day, so let your body do what it needs to heal and recover.

25DAYS

Another reason these days are so essential is that they will tell you how you're progressing. For me, my rest days are my first indicator that I'm accomplishing my goals. Because if I'm not coming back to my workouts in pain, feeling less invigorated, and lacking resolve to continue working toward my goals, then I'm already successful before I see any physical progress in my workout.

The fact is, before you start seeing changes in your performance and physique—before you begin noticing that you can run faster, jump higher, lift more weight, or any improvement in any of those typically measured outcomes—you'll discover you'll start recovering from your workouts much faster and feel more energized

That's why I want you to take these days seriously. If you doubt that what you're doing is working and you want another way to measure if you're getting in shape, then gauge how you feel after each Secondary Day 3. Do you come back the next day feeling like you can take over the world—or do you still feel tired and miserable? I can guarantee that if you take the time to compare how you feel after each Secondary Day 3, you'll notice an immediate difference in how much better you feel and how motivated you are.

IF you're looking for something else to do . . .

THEN try a yoga class.

I don't mind you substituting an hour-long session of low-intensity yoga that day, so long as it's not one of the high-intensity forms such as vinyasa, ashtanga, or power yoga. The overly vigorous styles tend to be too stressful and won't allow your muscles or central nervous system enough time to heal. Instead, choose more passive styles such as restorative, yin, kundalini, and viniyoga, which help stretch your muscles as opposed to strengthening them.

MOVING MEDITATION

(THE STRETCHES)

1. STANDING QUAD STRETCH (LOOSENS THE QUADRICEPS)

- ✦ **Start position:** Stand with your feet shoulder width apart and your arms down at your sides. Bend your right leg to bring your right foot back directly behind you and grab it with your left hand. You should immediately feel a gentle stretch along the front of your thigh.

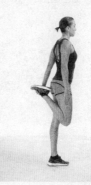

- ✦ **How to do it:** Gently pull your foot toward your body until you feel a comfortable stretch. Hold for 2 or 3 breaths, return your foot to the floor, and then repeat the stretch with your left leg.

IF you have a hard time balancing on one foot . . .

THEN use only one hand to grab your foot and use the other to hold on to something for balance.

2. MODIFIED FLANK (stretches the spine)

- ✦ **Start position:** Stand with your right foot about 3 feet in front of your left foot, your arms down by your sides.

- ✦ **How to do it:** Drop down into a lunge position so that your left knee touches the floor and your right leg is bent at a 90-degree

25DAYS

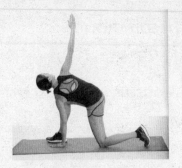

angle. Twist your torso to the right and extend your right arm straight up to the ceiling as you touch your left hand to the floor. Open up your body so that your chest faces the side as you turn your head to look upward. Hold for 2 or 3 breaths and then switch positions—left foot forward, right foot back, twisting to your left this time—to repeat the stretch.

IF you can't twist far enough at the waist . . .

THEN twist only as far as you comfortably can.

3. SINGLE-LEG HAMSTRING STRETCH (loosens the hamstrings and calves)

+ **Start position:** Sit on the floor with your legs extended in front of you. Bend your right leg and turn it inward so that your right foot rests against the inside of your left thigh.

+ **How to do it:** Reach toward your left foot with your left hand and grab your toes. Lean forward until you feel a comfortable stretch and then hold for 2 or 3 breaths. Switch positions to work the opposite leg.

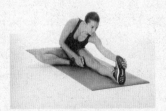

4. HALF LORD OF THE FISH POSE (stretches the hips, glutes, chest, shoulders, and neck)

✦ **Start position:** Sit on the floor with your legs straight in front of you. Bend your left leg and place your left foot flat on the floor just along the outside of your right knee.

✦ **How to do it:** Twisting at the waist, gently turn your body to the left and place your left hand flat on the floor behind you. Place your right elbow on the outside of your left knee. Look as far back over your left shoulder as you can comfortably. Hold for 2 or 3 breaths and then switch positions— left leg straight, right leg bent, twisting to your right this time—to repeat the stretch.

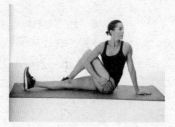

5. COBRA (stretches the core)

+ **Start position:** Lie facedown on the floor with your legs straight and your arms bent, with your hands placed flat on the floor alongside your shoulders. Position your feet so that you are resting on top of them; don't rise up on your toes.

+ **How to do it:** Keeping your legs flat on the floor, straighten your arms gently as you push your pelvis down and curl your torso up off the floor. Raise your chin up to the ceiling as far as you comfortably can and then hold at the top for 2 or 3 breaths. Slowly roll yourself back down into the start position.

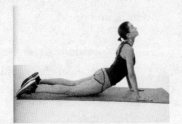

IF you can't straighten your arms completely . . .

THEN extend them as far as you comfortably can.

6. FEET OVER HEAD (stretches the lower back)

+ **Start position:** Lie on your back on a mat or carpeted surface with your legs straight and your arms down at your sides, palms facing the floor.

+ **How to do it:** Bend your knees and slowly bring your feet up and back over your head, keeping your hands flat on the floor. Try to extend your legs so that your toes touch the

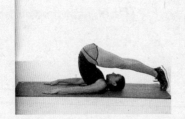

floor. If you're not that flexible, that's fine; just lower your feet as close to the floor as you can. Hold the stretch for 2 or 3 breaths and then slowly roll back down into the start position.

IF you can't get your legs all the way over your head . . .

THEN just pull up your knees toward your chest as far as you can. Place your hands on your knees and pull them gently toward your body.

chapter ten

....

The 25Days Daily Grading Sheets

This is it. This is where you'll succeed today. This is where you'll succeed tomorrow. This is where—in as few as twenty-five days—you'll make the neurological changes that will allow you to succeed for the rest of your life.

Here you'll find twenty-five daily grading sheets—one for each day—complete with how to grade yourself when it comes to each meal and snack, as well as your exercise requirements for the day. The rules are simple:

EVERY DAY

+ Circle each percentage when you succeed, tally up your diet and exercise grades, and then add them both together.

+ Add to that grade any bonus points you may have earned that day.

+ Write your Cumulative Grade at the bottom of the sheet.

+ **Strive to make every Cumulative Grade 85 percent or higher!**

EVERY FIVE DAYS

+ You'll also find a grading sheet after the end of each 5-Day Block.

+ On this sheet, you'll write down your Cumulative Grades from your last five days, add them together, divide by 5, and write down your Block Grade.

- **Again, strive to make every Block Grade 85 percent or higher!**

AT THE END OF TWENTY-FIVE DAYS

- You'll find a final grading sheet at the very end.

- On this sheet, write down all five Block Grades that you received, add them together, divide by 5, and write down your Final Grade.

- **Again, strive to make your Final Grade 85 percent or higher!**

***IF** you find it hard to sleep while on the program . . .*

***THEN** tally up your grade after dinner instead of later at night.*

Researchers from the Center for Biomedical Research in Neuro-degenerative Diseases Network (CIBERNED) in Madrid and from the Faculty of Biology at the University of Barcelona found[*] that dopamine can inhibit the effects of norepinephrine, a hormone involved in regulating the brain's synthesis of melatonin, the hormone that helps control your sleep and wake cycles. According to their study, dopamine receptors show up in the brain's pineal gland only at the end of the night; therefore, it could be possible that experiencing a dopamine surge close to bedtime could decrease melatonin production, making sleep harder to come by.

---

*S. González et al., "Circadian-Related Heteromerization of Adrenergic and Dopamine D_4 Receptors Modulates Melatonin Synthesis and Release in the Pineal Gland," *PLoS Biol* 10, no. 6 (June 19, 2012): e1001347, doi:10.1371/journal.pbio.1001347.

BONUS POINTS–AND BRAIN PENALTIES!

Even though calculating your total score each day is as simple as adding up your meals and snacks, as well as scoring your performance when exercising, there are ways to either improve or reduce your daily score by making smarter choices or mistakes along the way. I mentioned a few throughout the book, but here they all are in one place, along with a few others that may help you make the most of the program:

Bonus Points

◆ If you drank 2 glasses of water—at least 24 ounces total—with *every* meal and every snack: add 1 point to your **daily** total grade.

◆ If you got a solid 7 to 8 hours of restful sleep: add 1 point to your **daily** total grade.

◆ If you performed your workout first thing in the morning immediately after waking up on an empty stomach: add 1 point to your **daily** total grade.

◆ If you ate nothing but strictly organic foods at every meal and snack: add 1 point to your **daily** total grade.

◆ If you measured out all your food to the gram: add 1 point to your **daily** total grade.

◆ If you prepared all of your meals and snacks, as opposed to eating out: add 1 point to your **daily** total grade.

Brain Penalties

◆ If you **cheated on a Primary Day:** deduct **20** percent from your total **daily nutrition grade** per serving.

◆ If you **cheated on a Secondary Day:** deduct **25** percent from your total **daily nutrition grade** per serving.

◆ If you **skipped an entire meal or snack:** you earn **0** percent for that meal or snack.

> ✦ If you **reached for anything but what I'm asking you to eat:** you earn **0** percent for that meal or snack.

BEFORE YOU START

When I work with clients one-on-one, instead of just telling them what to do, I want them to know what's happening with their bodies so that they know what to watch out for on certain days along the way. I want them to know what's normal and what to expect during each of the five 5-Day Blocks.

Not knowing how you may feel physically, mentally, and emotionally is one of the missing links in many workouts. It's like being given directions from point A to point B but never being told about the highs and lows you may run into in between. That's why if you're curious about what to expect as you go along, the next few pages will reveal a few landmarks you might expect to see—or any sudden turns.

You see, even though you're only alternating among the same five workouts, they will feel different each time you do them, depending on where they fall. I know when you'll feel more motivated and more energized. I also know when you're more likely to feel less motivated and more likely to try to phone it in.

If you don't mind surprises along the way, just go right to the Daily Grading Sheets on page 211 and get started! Otherwise, if you're curious about what makes each of the 5-Day Blocks special—and what to expect so you can better prepare for even greater results—here's what you need to know.

The 25Days Routine *Magnified*!

Block 1 (A1B2A)

In this 5-day block, you'll be doing three strength days with an emphasis on the lower-body muscles. That's because you'll be working your legs on Day 1 and Day 5, while challenging your upper body only on Day 3. The emphasis will also be on evoking a greater central nervous system response through the agility and coordination movements you'll be performing on Days 1 and 5 that will challenge your balance.

Block 1 is going to be the hardest for several reasons. First, of the two types of strength-training days, Primary Day A is harder than Primary Day B due to the exercises involved. So, since you'll be doing two Primary Day A's within the same block, it makes the block naturally more difficult but worthwhile to your muscles. It also has the two most difficult conditioning days of the three (Secondary Days 1 and 2).

A lot of well-designed programs typically start out harder in the beginning for a reason: most people are more dedicated when they first undertake a program. That's why some trainers (including me) typically don't start their clients off at *too* slow a pace and *then* build them up. The idea behind this first block is to shock your body toward the change that we want it to respond to.

What to Watch For. Expect that you'll feel more sore and exhausted than you will in subsequent blocks throughout the program. The reason: it's your first time, so there's a bit of a shock factor involved. It's also the most intense block. So when you combine that higher intensity and newness, there's an adage that says: "The best thing to do is the thing you're not doing." Anytime you take on a new program, regardless of whether you are a beginner or advanced exerciser, if it's something you've never done before or haven't done in a long time, you will naturally be more sore and tired than usual.

The Right Mind-set. Forget about perfection—focus on completion. As you begin to acclimate to the exercises in this first block, you'll be busy changing certain moves to make a few exercises easier or more difficult, as well as dealing with a higher concentration of lactic acid within your muscles. That's why I'm not looking to have you break any records when it comes to the time of your strength-training workouts. Instead, I want you to focus on maintaining a full, robust range of motion and just complete each workout, so you earn 100 percent.

Block 2 (3B1A2)

You're probably a little sore from Block 1—and that's okay. You'll be dialing back your strength-training sessions by one day during this 5-Day Block and adding in a restorative cardio day. So instead of having five intense days, you'll be dealing with only four.

The second block starts off with an active rest day that will allow your body time to recover and heal so that it can bounce back and be ready to go again. This active recovery day is going to promote healing, decrease soreness, flush out lactic acid, drain your lymph system, increase circulation, and help loosen up tightness in certain key muscle groups.

What to Watch For. At the end of Block 1, you'll be enjoying for the first time an **Every-Five-Day Mind Meal,** a carb-rich dinner your body will need to prevent it from slipping into starvation mode and to rebalance your brain chemistry.

On the positive side, having this meal the night before is going to significantly help your body heal and recover on Day 6. On the negative side—and it's nothing to be alarmed about, because it's natural for this to occur in some people—but you might wake up feeling a little swollen or bloated, depending on how sensitive you might be to carbohydrates. It's different for everybody, and I've found that certain clients are more reactive to this than others.

The thing to realize is that the bloat you're experiencing is all water—it's not fat. More important, even though you might not like how it looks on you temporarily, that extra water is helping along the healing process, working behind the scenes to flush out your system and the lactic acid within your muscles.

The Right Mind-set. Don't fight the bloat—boost it! I recommend that at the start of Block 2 you stay hydrated as much as possible. Even though it may seem counterproductive to drink more water when you may be experiencing a little bloating, it helps to circulate all of the extra glycogen and water that you'll be consuming during your Every-Five-Day Mind Meal. I want both to flush your system, and the more water you can drink, the better that process will take place.

DAYS 11 THROUGH 15

Block 3 (B3A1B)

This block is almost as intense as Block 1 because it also contains three strength-building days. However, two of the three strength-training days are focused on your upper body, using exercises that aren't as taxing on the central nervous system as the moves used for the lower body.

Early in Block 3, you're also going to have another active rest day on Day 12. But then you'll be jumping right back into the hardest strength-training day and hardest conditioning day back-to-back (Days 13 and 14). Having that active rest day will allow you to hit those two workouts fresh and unencumbered by lack of energy or soreness, so don't be surprised if you notice a big improvement in your performance from when you tackled them back-to-back on Days 1 and 2.

What to Watch For. If you're female and it's your first time undertaking a strength-training program, or it's been a while since you've done one, don't be surprised if you're not able to maintain the same intensity on Day 15 as you did on Day 11, the reason being, typically—but not necessarily across the board—that women's upper bodies aren't as resilient as men's are. So you might experience more soreness than usual from not spending as much time focusing on the upper body as you might on the lower half.

The Right Mind-set. Just go—and expect to be slow. I don't want you feeling guilty and thinking that you're somehow failing by not being as up-tempo on Day 15. The thing I always tell my clients, and now share with you, is that your muscles can't count, and your muscles can't measure. All they know is what's hard and what's not. So as long as you're pushing yourself with the same amount of effort, don't beat yourself up over the time. Just complete it and get that grade.

DAYS 16 THROUGH 20

Block 4 (2A3B1)

Block 4 is my favorite, and here's why: you have to strength train only two days out of the five, your active recovery day falls right dead center, and your hardest conditioning day is saved until the very end. This is the block where I find my clients finally saying, "Hey, I'm getting the hang of this!"

What to Watch For. I predict that on Day 17, the second day of this block, you'll experience the best Primary Day A workout you've had up until this point as far as how quickly you perform it, how many reps and rounds you're able to do, and how quickly you recover. Why? Because your body has begun to acclimate to what's happening to it. And, when paired with the cumulative effects of eating three **Every-Five-Day Mind Meals**—in addition to eating better in general over the last several weeks—any soreness that might have lingered should be gone.

The Right Mind-set. Let success go to your head. What I mean by that is, I want you to be proud of yourself for reaching this point, so go right ahead and give yourself a big pat on the back. But more important, I want you to use this week as proof that what you're doing is having the right effect on both your body and your brain. The more you can get yourself to trust the plan, the longer you'll stick it out to ensure that you're rewiring your brain and creating the new neurological patterns you're trying to.

25DAYS

Block 5 (A2B3A)

If this one looks familiar, it should, because you're practically right back at the start. During this final block, you'll be following the same type of strength-training schedule you performed on the very first block. The only difference: you'll be taking it a little easier on your Secondary Days, and you'll have an active recovery day close to the very end.

What to Watch For. At this point, you'll have put in a significant amount of time running the nutrition and workout programs in concert with each other. Because of this, your body should have started to create a rhythm where it expects what's coming, whether it's a strength-training day, a conditioning day, or an active rest day.

That's why this is when I typically find my clients to be most alert and motivated, so expect your energy levels to be high. Also, your mind will be wrapped around knowing you're at the end of the program and about to receive your first Total Grade, so this block feels almost like you're taking the finals. It's when everybody typically gears up and pushes to do his or her best.

This is also when I find that most clients are the most solid with their diets and feel good about every single exercise. It's also around the time you should begin noticing that you're looking a little better. It's when your friends start telling you that something seems different about you, even if you don't see those changes yourself just yet.

The Right Mind-set. Make this block your measuring stick. If you haven't truly pushed yourself up until now, I want you to go for it. This is your opportunity to really see what your hard work from Block 1 to Block 5 has added up to. By comparing the results of both blocks— looking at how many reps and rounds you were able to complete at first and seeing how much faster you've become at achieving them now— you'll have actual evidence of how much stronger and better conditioned you are, because you are doing the same exact program (for the most part) as in Block 1.

Your Daily Grading Sheets

BREAKFAST   20%
F: 30 g. protein/20 g. fibrous carbs/10 g. fat/glass water
M: 40 g. protein/30 g. fibrous carbs/15 g. fat/glass water

SNACK   20%
F: 15 g. protein/10 g. fibrous carbs/5 g. fat/glass water
M: 20 g. protein/15 g. fibrous carbs/7.5 g. fat/glass water

LUNCH   20%
F: 30 g. protein/20 g. fibrous carbs/10 g. fat/glass water
M: 40 g. protein/30 g. fibrous carbs/15 g. fat/glass water

SNACK   20%
F: 15 g. protein/10 g. fibrous carbs/5 g. fat/glass water
M: 20 g. protein/15 g. fibrous carbs/7.5 g. fat/glass water

DINNER   20%
F: 30 g. protein/20 g. fibrous carbs/10 g. fat/glass water
M: 40 g. protein/30 g. fibrous carbs/15 g. fat/glass water

Total Diet____%

Primary Day A

1. Spartan Lunges
2. Rocking Horses
3. Plank-ups
4. Split Jump Squats
5. Modified Fire Hydrants
Jump rope for 30 seconds—then repeat the circuit for the required number of rounds.

Level	Reps	Rounds	Score per round (percent)
Beginner	5 to 8	3	33
Intermediate	8 to 12	4	25
Advanced	12 to 15	5	20

(Time:_____:_____)

Total Exercise____%

TOTAL DIET AND EXERCISE_____%
Bonus Points_____%

CUMULATIVE GRADE _____%

BREAKFAST 20%
F: 30 g. protein/20 g. fibrous carbs/10 g. fat/glass water
M: 40 g. protein/30 g. fibrous carbs/15 g. fat/glass water

LUNCH 20%
F: 30 g. protein/20 g. fibrous carbs/10 g. fat/glass water
M: 40 g. protein/30 g. fibrous carbs/15 g. fat/glass water

SNACK 20%
F: 15 g. protein/10 g. fibrous carbs/5 g. fat/glass water
M: 20 g. protein/15 g. fibrous carbs/7.5 g. fat/glass water

DINNER 20%
F: 30 g. protein/20 g. fibrous carbs/10 g. fat/glass water
M: 40 g. protein/30 g. fibrous carbs/15 g. fat/glass water

Total Diet____%

Secondary Day 1

1. Burpees (8 reps)
2. Lateral Hops (20 reps total, 10 each side)
3. High Knee Sprints (20 reps total, 10 each leg)
4. Alternating Donkey Kicks (20 reps total, 10 each leg)
5. Jumping Wood Chops (10 reps)
6. Single-Leg Thrusters (10 reps total, 5 each side)
Toe Taps for 30 seconds—then repeat the circuit for the required number of rounds.

Level	Rounds	Score per round (percent)
Beginner	3	33
Intermediate	4	25
Advanced	5	20

Total Exercise____%

TOTAL DIET AND EXERCISE____%
Bonus Points____%

CUMULATIVE GRADE _____%

BREAKFAST	20%

F: 30 g. protein/20 g. fibrous carbs/10 g. fat/glass water
M: 40 g. protein/30 g. fibrous carbs/15 g. fat/glass water

SNACK	20%

F: 15 g. protein/10 g. fibrous carbs/5 g. fat/glass water
M: 20 g. protein/15 g. fibrous carbs/7.5 g. fat/glass water

LUNCH	20%

F: 30 g. protein/20 g. fibrous carbs/10 g. fat/glass water
M: 40 g. protein/30 g. fibrous carbs/15 g. fat/glass water

SNACK	20%

F: 15 g. protein/10 g. fibrous carbs/5 g. fat/glass water
M: 20 g. protein/15 g. fibrous carbs/7.5 g. fat/glass water

DINNER	20%

F: 30 g. protein/20 g. fibrous carbs/10 g. fat/glass water
M: 40 g. protein/30 g. fibrous carbs/15 g. fat/glass water

Total Diet____%

Primary Day B

1. Push-ups
2. Standing Band Rows
3. Hop Squats
4. Seated Dips
5. Upright Row/Curls
Jump rope for 30 seconds—then repeat the circuit for the required number of rounds.

Level	Reps	Rounds	Score per round (percent)
Beginner	5 to 8	3	33
Intermediate	8 to 12	4	25
Advanced	12 to 15	5	20

(Time:_____:_____)

Total Exercise____%

TOTAL DIET AND EXERCISE_____%
Bonus Points_____%

CUMULATIVE GRADE _____%

BREAKFAST   25%
F: 30 g. protein/20 g. fibrous carbs/10 g. fat/glass water
M: 40 g. protein/30 g. fibrous carbs/15 g. fat/glass water

LUNCH   25%
F: 30 g. protein/20 g. fibrous carbs/10 g. fat/glass water
M: 40 g. protein/30 g. fibrous carbs/15 g. fat/glass water

SNACK   25%
F: 15 g. protein/10 g. fibrous carbs/5 g. fat/glass water
M: 20 g. protein/15 g. fibrous carbs/7.5 g. fat/glass water

DINNER   25%
F: 30 g. protein/20 g. fibrous carbs/10 g. fat/glass water
M: 40 g. protein/30 g. fibrous carbs/15 g. fat/glass water

Total Diet____%

Secondary Day 2

Pick any 3 exercises and create your own circuit, but include at least 1 exercise with an asterisk.

1. *Burpees (8 reps)
2. Lateral Hops (20 reps total, 10 each side)
3. *High Knee Sprints (20 reps total, 10 each leg)
4. Alternating Donkey Kicks (20 reps total, 10 each leg)
5. *Jumping Wood Chops (10 reps)
6. Single-Leg Thrusters (10 reps total, 5 each side)

Toe Taps for 30 seconds—then repeat the circuit for the required number of rounds.

Level	Rounds	Score per round (percent)
Beginner	3	33
Intermediate	4	25
Advanced	5	20

Total Exercise____ %

TOTAL DIET AND EXERCISE____ %
Bonus Points____ %

CUMULATIVE GRADE _____ %

| | | |
| | | |

BREAKFAST   20%
F: 30 g. protein/20 g. fibrous carbs/10 g. fat/glass water
M: 40 g. protein/30 g. fibrous carbs/15 g. fat/glass water

SNACK   20%
F: 15 g. protein/10 g. fibrous carbs/5 g. fat/glass water
M: 20 g. protein/15 g. fibrous carbs/7.5 g. fat/glass water

LUNCH   20%
F: 30 g. protein/20 g. fibrous carbs/10 g. fat/glass water
M: 40 g. protein/30 g. fibrous carbs/15 g. fat/glass water

SNACK   20%
F: 15 g. protein/10 g. fibrous carbs/5 g. fat/glass water
M: 20 g. protein/15 g. fibrous carbs/7.5 g. fat/glass water

EVERY 5-DAY MIND MEAL (DINNER)   20%
F: no more than 80 g. low-glycemic starchy carbs/glass water
M: no more than 120 g. low-glycemic starchy carbs/glass water

Total Diet____ %

Primary Day A

1. Spartan Lunges
2. Rocking Horses
3. Plank-ups
4. Split Jump Squats
5. Modified Fire Hydrants
Jump rope for 30 seconds—then repeat the circuit for the required number of rounds.

	Reps	Rounds	Score per round (percent)
Beginner	5 to 8	3	33
Intermediate	8 to 12	4	25
Advanced	12 to 15	5	20

(Time:_____:_____)

Total Exercise____ %

TOTAL DIET AND EXERCISE_____ %
Bonus Points_____ %

CUMULATIVE GRADE _____ %

Cumulative Grade Day 1_____ %

Cumulative Grade Day 2_____ %

Cumulative Grade Day 3_____ %

Cumulative Grade Day 4_____ %

Cumulative Grade Day 5_____ %

1ST BLOCK GRADE_____ %

BREAKFAST   25%
F: 30 g. protein/20 g. fibrous carbs/10 g. fat/glass water
M: 40 g. protein/30 g. fibrous carbs/15 g. fat/glass water

LUNCH   25%
F: 30 g. protein/20 g. fibrous carbs/10 g. fat/glass water
M: 40 g. protein/30 g. fibrous carbs/15 g. fat/glass water

SNACK   25%
F: 15 g. protein/10 g. fibrous carbs/5 g. fat/glass water
M: 20 g. protein/15 g. fibrous carbs/7.5 g. fat/glass water

DINNER   25%
F: 30 g. protein/20 g. fibrous carbs/10 g. fat/glass water
M: 40 g. protein/30 g. fibrous carbs/15 g. fat/glass water

Total Diet____ %

Secondary Day 3

Perform a low-intensity activity for a minimum of 30 minutes *and* the Moving Meditation circuit to earn 100 percent.
1. Standing Quad Stretch
2. Modified Flank
3. Single-Leg Hamstring Stretch
4. Half Lord of the Fish Pose
5. Cobra
6. Feet over Head
Hold each stretch for a minimum of 30 seconds—repeat the circuit for 3 rounds. Give yourself an extra 5 percent if you do 4 rounds; 10 percent if you do 5 rounds.

Bonus Points____%

Total Exercise____ %

TOTAL DIET AND EXERCISE_____ %
Bonus Points_____ %

CUMULATIVE GRADE _____ %

BREAKFAST 20%
F: 30 g. protein/20 g. fibrous carbs/10 g. fat/glass water
M: 40 g. protein/30 g. fibrous carbs/15 g. fat/glass water

SNACK 20%
F: 15 g. protein/10 g. fibrous carbs/5 g. fat/glass water
M: 20 g. protein/15 g. fibrous carbs/7.5 g. fat/glass water

LUNCH 20%
F: 30 g. protein/20 g. fibrous carbs/10 g. fat/glass water
M: 40 g. protein/30 g. fibrous carbs/15 g. fat/glass water

SNACK 20%
F: 15 g. protein/10 g. fibrous carbs/5 g. fat/glass water
M: 20 g. protein/15 g. fibrous carbs/7.5 g. fat/glass water

DINNER 20%
F: 30 g. protein/20 g. fibrous carbs/10 g. fat/glass water
M: 40 g. protein/30 g. fibrous carbs/15 g. fat/glass water

Total Diet____ %

1. Push-ups
2. Standing Band Rows
3. Hop Squats
4. Seated Dips
5. Upright Row/Curls

Jump rope for 30 seconds—then repeat the circuit for the required number of rounds.

Level	Reps	Rounds	Score per round (percent)
Beginner	5 to 8	3	33
Intermediate	8 to 12	4	25
Advanced	12 to 15	5	20

(Time:_____:_____)

Total Exercise____%

TOTAL DIET AND EXERCISE_____ %
Bonus Points_____ %

CUMULATIVE GRADE _____ %

DREW LOGAN

BREAKFAST   25%
F: 30 g. protein/20 g. fibrous carbs/10 g. fat/glass water
M: 40 g. protein/30 g. fibrous carbs/15 g. fat/glass water

LUNCH   25%
F: 30 g. protein/20 g. fibrous carbs/10 g. fat/glass water
M: 40 g. protein/30 g. fibrous carbs/15 g. fat/glass water

SNACK   25%
F: 15 g. protein/10 g. fibrous carbs/5 g. fat/glass water
M: 20 g. protein/15 g. fibrous carbs/7.5 g. fat/glass water

DINNER   25%
F: 30 g. protein/20 g. fibrous carbs/10 g. fat/glass water
M: 40 g. protein/30 g. fibrous carbs/15 g. fat/glass water

Total Diet____ %

Secondary Day 1

1. Burpees (8 reps)
2. Lateral Hops (20 reps total, 10 each side)
3. High Knee Sprints (20 reps total, 10 each leg)
4. Alternating Donkey Kicks (20 reps total, 10 each leg)
5. Jumping Wood Chops (10 reps)
6. Single-Leg Thrusters (10 reps total, 5 each side)
Toe Taps for 30 seconds—then repeat the circuit for the required number of rounds.

Level	Rounds	Score per round (percent)
Beginner	3	33
Intermediate	4	25
Advanced	5	20

Total Exercise____ %

TOTAL DIET AND EXERCISE_____ %
Bonus Points_____ %

CUMULATIVE GRADE _____ %

BREAKFAST 20%
F: 30 g. protein/20 g. fibrous carbs/10 g. fat/glass water
M: 40 g. protein/30 g. fibrous carbs/15 g. fat/glass water

SNACK 20%
F: 15 g. protein/10 g. fibrous carbs/5 g. fat/glass water
M: 20 g. protein/15 g. fibrous carbs/7.5 g. fat/glass water

LUNCH 20%
F: 30 g. protein/20 g. fibrous carbs/10 g. fat/glass water
M: 40 g. protein/30 g. fibrous carbs/15 g. fat/glass water

SNACK 20%
F: 15 g. protein/10 g. fibrous carbs/5 g. fat/glass water
M: 20 g. protein/15 g. fibrous carbs/7.5 g. fat/glass water

DINNER 20%
F: 30 g. protein/20 g. fibrous carbs/10 g. fat/glass water
M: 40 g. protein/30 g. fibrous carbs/15 g. fat/glass water

Total Diet____ %

1. Spartan Lunges
2. Rocking Horses
3. Plank-ups
4. Split Jump Squats
5. Modified Fire Hydrants

Jump rope for 30 seconds—then repeat the circuit for the required number of rounds.

Level	Reps	Rounds	Score per round (percent)
Beginner	5 to 8	3	33
Intermediate	8 to 12	4	25
Advanced	12 to 15	5	20

(Time:____:____)

Total Exercise____ %

TOTAL DIET AND EXERCISE____ %
Bonus Points____ %

CUMULATIVE GRADE ____ %

BREAKFAST 25%
F: 30 g. protein/20 g. fibrous carbs/10 g. fat/glass water
M: 40 g. protein/30 g. fibrous carbs/15 g. fat/glass water

LUNCH 25%
F: 30 g. protein/20 g. fibrous carbs/10 g. fat/glass water
M: 40 g. protein/30 g. fibrous carbs/15 g. fat/glass water

SNACK 25%
F: 15 g. protein/10 g. fibrous carbs/5 g. fat/glass water
M: 20 g. protein/15 g. fibrous carbs/7.5 g. fat/glass water

EVERY 5-DAY MIND MEAL (DINNER) 25%
F: no more than 80 g. low-glycemic starchy carbs/glass water
M: no more than 120 g. low-glycemic starchy carbs/glass water

Total Diet____ %

Secondary Day 2

Pick any 3 exercises and create your own circuit, but include at least 1 exercise with an asterisk.
1. *Burpees (8 reps)
2. Lateral Hops (20 reps total, 10 each side)
3. *High Knee Sprints (20 reps total, 10 each leg)
4. Alternating Donkey Kicks (20 reps total, 10 each leg)
5. *Jumping Wood Chops (10 reps)
6. Single-Leg Thrusters (10 reps total, 5 each side)
Toe Taps for 30 seconds—then repeat the circuit for the required number of rounds.

Level	Rounds	Score per round (percent)
Beginner	3	33
Intermediate	4	25
Advanced	5	20

Total Exercise____ %

TOTAL DIET AND EXERCISE_____ %
Bonus Points_____ %

CUMULATIVE GRADE _____ %

Cumulative Grade Day 6_____ %

Cumulative Grade Day 7_____ %

Cumulative Grade Day 8_____ %

Cumulative Grade Day 9_____ %

Cumulative Grade Day 10_____ %

2ND BLOCK GRADE_____ %

BREAKFAST   20%
F: 30 g. protein/20 g. fibrous carbs/10 g. fat/glass water
M: 40 g. protein/30 g. fibrous carbs/15 g. fat/glass water

SNACK   20%
F: 15 g. protein/10 g. fibrous carbs/5 g. fat/glass water
M: 20 g. protein/15 g. fibrous carbs/7.5 g. fat/glass water

LUNCH   20%
F: 30 g. protein/20 g. fibrous carbs/10 g. fat/glass water
M: 40 g. protein/30 g. fibrous carbs/15 g. fat/glass water

SNACK   20%
F: 15 g. protein/10 g. fibrous carbs/5 g. fat/glass water
M: 20 g. protein/15 g. fibrous carbs/7.5 g. fat/glass water

DINNER   20%
F: 30 g. protein/20 g. fibrous carbs/10 g. fat/glass water
M: 40 g. protein/30 g. fibrous carbs/15 g. fat/glass water

Total Diet____ %

Primary Day B

1. Push-ups
2. Standing Band Rows
3. Hop Squats
4. Seated Dips
5. Upright Row/Curls

Jump rope for 30 seconds—then repeat the circuit for the required number of rounds.

Level	Reps	Rounds	Score per round (percent)
Beginner	5 to 8	3	33
Intermediate	8 to 12	4	25
Advanced	12 to 15	5	20

(Time:_____:_____)

Total Exercise____ %

TOTAL DIET AND EXERCISE_____ %
Bonus Points_____ %

          CUMULATIVE GRADE _____ %

BREAKFAST   25%
F: 30 g. protein/20 g. fibrous carbs/10 g. fat/glass water
M: 40 g. protein/30 g. fibrous carbs/15 g. fat/glass water

LUNCH   25%
F: 30 g. protein/20 g. fibrous carbs/10 g. fat/glass water
M: 40 g. protein/30 g. fibrous carbs/15 g. fat/glass water

SNACK   25%
F: 15 g. protein/10 g. fibrous carbs/5 g. fat/glass water
M: 20 g. protein/15 g. fibrous carbs/7.5 g. fat/glass water

DINNER   25%
F: 30 g. protein/20 g. fibrous carbs/10 g. fat/glass water
M: 40 g. protein/30 g. fibrous carbs/15 g. fat/glass water

Total Diet____ %

Secondary Day 3

Perform a low-intensity activity for a minimum of 30 minutes *and* the Moving Meditation circuit to earn 100 percent.
1. Standing Quad Stretch
2. Modified Flank
3. Single-Leg Hamstring Stretch
4. Half Lord of the Fish Pose
5. Cobra
6. Feet over Head

Hold each stretch for a minimum of 30 seconds; repeat the circuit for 3 rounds. Give yourself an extra 5 percent if you do 4 rounds; 10 percent if you do 5 rounds.

Bonus Points____ %

Total Exercise____ %

TOTAL DIET AND EXERCISE_____ %
Bonus Points_____ %

CUMULATIVE GRADE _____ %

BREAKFAST   20%
F: 30 g. protein/20 g. fibrous carbs/10 g. fat/glass water
M: 40 g. protein/30 g. fibrous carbs/15 g. fat/glass water

SNACK   20%
F: 15 g. protein/10 g. fibrous carbs/5 g. fat/glass water
M: 20 g. protein/15 g. fibrous carbs/7.5 g. fat/glass water

LUNCH   20%
F: 30 g. protein/20 g. fibrous carbs/10 g. fat/glass water
M: 40 g. protein/30 g. fibrous carbs/15 g. fat/glass water

SNACK   20%
F: 15 g. protein/10 g. fibrous carbs/5 g. fat/glass water
M: 20 g. protein/15 g. fibrous carbs/7.5 g. fat/glass water

DINNER   20%
F: 30 g. protein/20 g. fibrous carbs/10 g. fat/glass water
M: 40 g. protein/30 g. fibrous carbs/15 g. fat/glass water

Total Diet____ %

Primary Day A

1. Spartan Lunges
2. Rocking Horses
3. Plank-ups
4. Split Jump Squats
5. Modified Fire Hydrants

Jump rope for 30 seconds—then repeat the circuit for the required number of rounds.

Level	Reps	Rounds	Score per round (percent)
Beginner	5 to 8	3	33
Intermediate	8 to 12	4	25
Advanced	12 to 15	5	20

(Time:_____:_____)

Total Exercise____ %

TOTAL DIET AND EXERCISE_____ %
Bonus Points_____ %

CUMULATIVE GRADE _____ %

BREAKFAST   25%
F: 30 g. protein/20 g. fibrous carbs/10 g. fat/glass water
M: 40 g. protein/30 g. fibrous carbs/15 g. fat/glass water

LUNCH   25%
F: 30 g. protein/20 g. fibrous carbs/10 g. fat/glass water
M: 40 g. protein/30 g. fibrous carbs/15 g. fat/glass water

SNACK   25%
F: 15 g. protein/10 g. fibrous carbs/5 g. fat/glass water
M: 20 g. protein/15 g. fibrous carbs/7.5 g. fat/glass water

DINNER   25%
F: 30 g. protein/20 g. fibrous carbs/10 g. fat/glass water
M: 40 g. protein/30 g. fibrous carbs/15 g. fat/glass water

Total Diet____ %

Secondary Day 1

1. Burpees (8 reps)
2. Lateral Hops (20 reps total, 10 each side)
3. High Knee Sprints (20 reps total, 10 each leg)
4. Alternating Donkey Kicks (20 reps total, 10 each leg)
5. Jumping Wood Chops (10 reps)
6. Single-Leg Thrusters (10 reps total, 5 each side)
Toe Taps for 30 seconds—then repeat the circuit for the required number of rounds.

Level	Rounds	Score per round (percent)
Beginner	3	33
Intermediate	4	25
Advanced	5	20

Total Exercise____ %

TOTAL DIET AND EXERCISE_____ %
Bonus Points_____ %

CUMULATIVE GRADE _____ %

BREAKFAST   20%
F: 30 g. protein/20 g. fibrous carbs/10 g. fat/glass water
M: 40 g. protein/30 g. fibrous carbs/15 g. fat/glass water

SNACK   20%
F: 15 g. protein/10 g. fibrous carbs/5 g. fat/glass water
M: 20 g. protein/15 g. fibrous carbs/7.5 g. fat/glass water

LUNCH   20%
F: 30 g. protein/20 g. fibrous carbs/10 g. fat/glass water
M: 40 g. protein/30 g. fibrous carbs/15 g. fat/glass water

SNACK   20%
F: 15 g. protein/10 g. fibrous carbs/5 g. fat/glass water
M: 20 g. protein/15 g. fibrous carbs/7.5 g. fat/glass water

EVERY-FIVE-DAY MIND MEAL (DINNER)   20%
F: no more than 80 g. low-glycemic starchy carbs/glass water
M: no more than 120 g. low-glycemic starchy carbs/glass water

Total Diet____ %

Primary Day B

1. Push-ups
2. Standing Band Rows
3. Hop Squats
4. Seated Dips
5. Upright Row/Curls
Jump rope for 30 seconds—then repeat the circuit for the required number of rounds.

Level	Reps	Rounds	Score per round (percent)
Beginner	5 to 8	3	33
Intermediate	8 to 12	4	25
Advanced	12 to 15	5	20

(Time:_____:_____)

Total Exercise____ %

TOTAL DIET AND EXERCISE_____ %
Bonus Points_____ %
               CUMULATIVE GRADE _____ %

Cumulative Grade Day 11_____ %

Cumulative Grade Day 12_____ %

Cumulative Grade Day 13_____ %

Cumulative Grade Day 14_____ %

Cumulative Grade Day 15_____ %

3RD BLOCK GRADE_____ %

BREAKFAST 25%
F: 30 g. protein/20 g. fibrous carbs/10 g. fat/glass water
M: 40 g. protein/30 g. fibrous carbs/15 g. fat/glass water

LUNCH 25%
F: 30 g. protein/20 g. fibrous carbs/10 g. fat/glass water
M: 40 g. protein/30 g. fibrous carbs/15 g. fat/glass water

SNACK 25%
F: 15 g. protein/10 g. fibrous carbs/5 g. fat/glass water
M: 20 g. protein/15 g. fibrous carbs/7.5 g. fat/glass water

DINNER 25%
F: 30 g. protein/20 g. fibrous carbs/10 g. fat/glass water
M: 40 g. protein/30 g. fibrous carbs/15 g. fat/glass water

Total Diet____ %

Secondary Day 2

Pick any 3 exercises and create your own circuit, but include at least 1 exercise with an asterisk.
1. *Burpees (8 reps)
2. Lateral Hops (20 reps total, 10 each side)
3. *High Knee Sprints (20 reps total, 10 each leg)
4. Alternating Donkey Kicks (20 reps total, 10 each leg)
5. *Jumping Wood Chops (10 reps)
6. Single-Leg Thrusters (10 reps total, 5 each side)
Toe Taps for 30 seconds—then repeat the circuit for the required number of rounds.

Level	Rounds	Score per round (percent)
Beginner	3	33
Intermediate	4	25
Advanced	5	20

Total Exercise____ %

TOTAL DIET AND EXERCISE____ %
Bonus Points____ %

CUMULATIVE GRADE _____ %

BREAKFAST 20%
F: 30 g. protein/20 g. fibrous carbs/10 g. fat/glass water
M: 40 g. protein/30 g. fibrous carbs/15 g. fat/glass water

SNACK 20%
F: 15 g. protein/10 g. fibrous carbs/5 g. fat/glass water
M: 20 g. protein/15 g. fibrous carbs/7.5 g. fat/glass water

LUNCH 20%
F: 30 g. protein/20 g. fibrous carbs/10 g. fat/glass water
M: 40 g. protein/30 g. fibrous carbs/15 g. fat/glass water

SNACK 20%
F: 15 g. protein/10 g. fibrous carbs/5 g. fat/glass water
M: 20 g. protein/15 g. fibrous carbs/7.5 g. fat/glass water

DINNER 20%
F: 30 g. protein/20 g. fibrous carbs/10 g. fat/glass water
M: 40 g. protein/30 g. fibrous carbs/15 g. fat/glass water

Total Diet____ %

Primary Day A

1. Spartan Lunges
2. Rocking Horses
3. Plank-ups
4. Split Jump Squats
5. Modified Fire Hydrants

Jump rope for 30 seconds—then repeat the circuit for the required number of rounds.

Level	Reps	Rounds	Score per round (percent)
Beginner	5 to 8	3	33
Intermediate	8 to 12	4	25
Advanced	12 to 15	5	20

(Time:_____:_____)

Total Exercise____ %

TOTAL DIET AND EXERCISE_____ %
Bonus Points_____ %

CUMULATIVE GRADE _____ %

....

BREAKFAST   25%
F: 30 g. protein/20 g. fibrous carbs/10 g. fat/glass water
M: 40 g. protein/30 g. fibrous carbs/15 g. fat/glass water

LUNCH   25%
F: 30 g. protein/20 g. fibrous carbs/10 g. fat/glass water
M: 40 g. protein/30 g. fibrous carbs/15 g. fat/glass water

SNACK   25%
F: 15 g. protein/10 g. fibrous carbs/5 g. fat/glass water
M: 20 g. protein/15 g. fibrous carbs/7.5 g. fat/glass water

DINNER   25%
F: 30 g. protein/20 g. fibrous carbs/10 g. fat/glass water
M: 40 g. protein/30 g. fibrous carbs/15 g. fat/glass water

Total Diet____%

....

Secondary Day 3

Perform a low-intensity activity for a minimum of 30 minutes *and* the Moving Meditation circuit to earn 100 percent.
1. Standing Quad Stretch
2. Modified Flank
3. Single-Leg Hamstring Stretch
4. Half Lord of the Fish Pose
5. Cobra
6. Feet over Head
Hold each stretch for a minimum of 30 seconds; repeat the circuit for 3 rounds. Give yourself an extra 5 percent if you do 4 rounds; 10 percent if you do 5 rounds.

Bonus Points____ %

Total Exercise____ %

TOTAL DIET AND EXERCISE_____ %
Bonus Points_____ %

CUMULATIVE GRADE _____ %

25DAYS

BREAKFAST   20%
F: 30 g. protein/20 g. fibrous carbs/10 g. fat/glass water
M: 40 g. protein/30 g. fibrous carbs/15 g. fat/glass water

SNACK   20%
F: 15 g. protein/10 g. fibrous carbs/5 g. fat/glass water
M: 20 g. protein/15 g. fibrous carbs/7.5 g. fat/glass water

LUNCH   20%
F: 30 g. protein/20 g. fibrous carbs/10 g. fat/glass water
M: 40 g. protein/30 g. fibrous carbs/15 g. fat/glass water

SNACK   20%
F: 15 g. protein/10 g. fibrous carbs/5 g. fat/glass water
M: 20 g. protein/15 g. fibrous carbs/7.5 g. fat/glass water

DINNER   20%
F: 30 g. protein/20 g. fibrous carbs/10 g. fat/glass water
M: 40 g. protein/30 g. fibrous carbs/15 g. fat/glass water

Total Diet____ %

Primary Day B

1. Push-ups
2. Standing Band Rows
3. Hop Squats
4. Seated Dips
5. Upright Row/Curls

Jump rope for 30 seconds—then repeat the circuit for the required number of rounds.

Level	Reps	Rounds	Score per round (percent)
Beginner	5 to 8	3	33
Intermediate	8 to 12	4	25
Advanced	12 to 15	5	20

(Time:_____:_____)

Total Exercise____ %

TOTAL DIET AND EXERCISE_____ %
Bonus Points_____ %

CUMULATIVE GRADE _____ %

BREAKFAST   25%
F: 30 g. protein/20 g. fibrous carbs/10 g. fat/glass water
M: 40 g. protein/30 g. fibrous carbs/15 g. fat/glass water

LUNCH   25%
F: 30 g. protein/20 g. fibrous carbs/10 g. fat/glass water
M: 40 g. protein/30 g. fibrous carbs/15 g. fat/glass water

SNACK   25%
F: 15 g. protein/10 g. fibrous carbs/5 g. fat/glass water
M: 20 g. protein/15 g. fibrous carbs/7.5 g. fat/glass water

EVERY-FIVE-DAY MIND MEAL (DINNER)   25%
F: no more than 80 g. low-glycemic starchy carbs/glass water
M: no more than 120 g. low-glycemic starchy carbs/glass water

Total Diet____ %

Secondary Day 1

1. Burpees (8 reps)
2. Lateral Hops (20 reps total, 10 each side)
3. High Knee Sprints (20 reps total, 10 each leg)
4. Alternating Donkey Kicks (20 reps total, 10 each leg)
5. Jumping Wood Chops (10 reps)
6. Single-Leg Thrusters (10 reps total, 5 each side)
Toe Taps for 30 seconds—then repeat the circuit for the required number
of rounds.

Level	Rounds	Score per round (percent)
Beginner	3	33
Intermediate	4	25
Advanced	5	20

Total Exercise____ %

TOTAL DIET AND EXERCISE_____ %
Bonus Points_____ %

CUMULATIVE GRADE _____ %

25DAYS

Cumulative Grade Day 16_____ %

Cumulative Grade Day 17_____ %

Cumulative Grade Day 18_____ %

Cumulative Grade Day 19_____ %

Cumulative Grade Day 20_____ %

4TH BLOCK GRADE_____ %

BREAKFAST   **20%**
F: 30 g. protein/20 g. fibrous carbs/10 g. fat/glass water
M: 40 g. protein/30 g. fibrous carbs/15 g. fat/glass water

SNACK   **20%**
F: 15 g. protein/10 g. fibrous carbs/5 g. fat/glass water
M: 20 g. protein/15 g. fibrous carbs/7.5 g. fat/glass water

LUNCH   **20%**
F: 30 g. protein/20 g. fibrous carbs/10 g. fat/glass water
M: 40 g. protein/30 g. fibrous carbs/15 g. fat/glass water

SNACK   **20%**
F: 15 g. protein/10 g. fibrous carbs/5 g. fat/glass water
M: 20 g. protein/15 g. fibrous carbs/7.5 g. fat/glass water

DINNER   **20%**
F: 30 g. protein/20 g. fibrous carbs/10 g. fat/glass water
M: 40 g. protein/30 g. fibrous carbs/15 g. fat/glass water

Total Diet____ %

Primary Day A

1. Spartan Lunges
2. Rocking Horses
3. Plank-ups
4. Split Jump Squats
5. Modified Fire Hydrants
Jump rope for 30 seconds—then repeat the circuit for the required number of rounds.

Level	Reps	Rounds	Score per round (percent)
Beginner	5 to 8	3	33
Intermediate	8 to 12	4	25
Advanced	12 to 15	5	20

(Time:_____:_____)

Total Exercise____ %

TOTAL DIET AND EXERCISE____ %
Bonus Points____ %

CUMULATIVE GRADE _____ %

BREAKFAST 25%
F: 30 g. protein/20 g. fibrous carbs/10 g. fat/glass water
M: 40 g. protein/30 g. fibrous carbs/15 g. fat/glass water

LUNCH 25%
F: 30 g. protein/20 g. fibrous carbs/10 g. fat/glass water
M: 40 g. protein/30 g. fibrous carbs/15 g. fat/glass water

SNACK 25%
F: 15 g. protein/10 g. fibrous carbs/5 g. fat/glass water
M: 20 g. protein/15 g. fibrous carbs/7.5 g. fat/glass water

DINNER 25%
F: 30 g. protein/20 g. fibrous carbs/10 g. fat/glass water
M: 40 g. protein/30 g. fibrous carbs/15 g. fat/glass water

Total Diet____ %

Secondary Day 2

Pick any 3 exercises and create your own circuit, but include at least 1 exercise with an asterisk.
1. *Burpees (8 reps)
2. Lateral Hops (20 reps total, 10 each side)
3. *High Knee Sprints (20 reps total, 10 each leg)
4. Alternating Donkey Kicks (20 reps total, 10 each leg)
5. *Jumping Wood Chops (10 reps)
6. Single-Leg Thrusters (10 reps total, 5 each side)
Toe Taps for 30 seconds—then repeat the circuit for the required number of rounds.

Level	Rounds	Score per round (percent)
Beginner	3	33
Intermediate	4	25
Advanced	5	20

Total Exercise____ %

TOTAL DIET AND EXERCISE____ %
Bonus Points____ %

CUMULATIVE GRADE ____ %

BREAKFAST   20%
F: 30 g. protein/20 g. fibrous carbs/10 g. fat/glass water
M: 40 g. protein/30 g. fibrous carbs/15 g. fat/glass water

SNACK   20%
F: 15 g. protein/10 g. fibrous carbs/5 g. fat/glass water
M: 20 g. protein/15 g. fibrous carbs/7.5 g. fat/glass water

LUNCH   20%
F: 30 g. protein/20 g. fibrous carbs/10 g. fat/glass water
M: 40 g. protein/30 g. fibrous carbs/15 g. fat/glass water

SNACK   20%
F: 15 g. protein/10 g. fibrous carbs/5 g. fat/glass water
M: 20 g. protein/15 g. fibrous carbs/7.5 g. fat/glass water

DINNER   20%
F: 30 g. protein/20 g. fibrous carbs/10 g. fat/glass water
M: 40 g. protein/30 g. fibrous carbs/15 g. fat/glass water

Total Diet____ %

Primary Day B

1. Push-ups
2. Standing Band Rows
3. Hop Squats
4. Seated Dips
5. Upright Row/Curls
Jump rope for 30 seconds—then repeat the circuit for the required number of rounds.

Level	Reps	Rounds	Score per round (percent)
Beginner	5 to 8	3	33
Intermediate	8 to 12	4	25
Advanced	12 to 15	5	20

(Time:_____:_____)

Total Exercise____ %

TOTAL DIET AND EXERCISE_____ %
Bonus Points_____ %

CUMULATIVE GRADE _____ %

BREAKFAST 25%
F: 30 g. protein/20 g. fibrous carbs/10 g. fat/glass water
M: 40 g. protein/30 g. fibrous carbs/15 g. fat/glass water

LUNCH 25%
F: 30 g. protein/20 g. fibrous carbs/10 g. fat/glass water
M: 40 g. protein/30 g. fibrous carbs/15 g. fat/glass water

SNACK 25%
F: 15 g. protein/10 g. fibrous carbs/5 g. fat/glass water
M: 20 g. protein/15 g. fibrous carbs/7.5 g. fat/glass water

DINNER 25%
F: 30 g. protein/20 g. fibrous carbs/10 g. fat/glass water
M: 40 g. protein/30 g. fibrous carbs/15 g. fat/glass water

Total Diet____ %

Secondary Day 3

Perform a low-intensity activity for a minimum of 30 minutes *and* the Moving Meditation circuit to earn 100%.
1. Standing Quad Stretch
2. Modified Flank
3. Single-Leg Hamstring Stretch
4. Half Lord of the Fish Pose
5. Cobra
6. Feet over Head
Hold each stretch for a minimum of 30 seconds; repeat the circuit for 3 rounds. Give yourself an extra 5 percent if you do 4 rounds; 10 percent if you do 5 rounds.

Bonus Points____ %

Total Exercise____ %

TOTAL DIET AND EXERCISE_____ %
Bonus Points_____ %

CUMULATIVE GRADE _____ %

BREAKFAST   20%
F: 30 g. protein/20 g. fibrous carbs/10 g. fat/glass water
M: 40 g. protein/30 g. fibrous carbs/15 g. fat/glass water

SNACK   20%
F: 15 g. protein/10 g. fibrous carbs/5 g. fat/glass water
M: 20 g. protein/15 g. fibrous carbs/7.5 g. fat/glass water

LUNCH   20%
F: 30 g. protein/20 g. fibrous carbs/10 g. fat/glass water
M: 40 g. protein/30 g. fibrous carbs/15 g. fat/glass water

SNACK   20%
F: 15 g. protein/10 g. fibrous carbs/5 g. fat/glass water
M: 20 g. protein/15 g. fibrous carbs/7.5 g. fat/glass water

EVERY-FIVE-DAY MIND MEAL (DINNER)   20%
F: no more than 80 g. low-glycemic starchy carbs/glass water
M: no more than 120 g. low-glycemic starchy carbs/glass water

Total Diet____ %

Primary Day A

1. Spartan Lunges
2. Rocking Horses
3. Plank-ups
4. Split Jump Squats
5. Modified Fire Hydrants
Jump rope for 30 seconds—then repeat the circuit for the required number of rounds.

Level	Reps	Rounds	Score per round (percent)
Beginner	5 to 8	3	33
Intermediate	8 to 12	4	25
Advanced	12 to 15	5	20

(Time:_____:_____)

Total Exercise____ %

TOTAL DIET AND EXERCISE_____ %
Bonus Points_____ %
                    CUMULATIVE GRADE _____ %

Cumulative Grade Day 21_____ %

Cumulative Grade Day 22_____ %

Cumulative Grade Day 23_____ %

Cumulative Grade Day 24_____ %

Cumulative Grade Day 25_____ %

5TH BLOCK GRADE_____ %

25DAYS FINAL GRADE

1st Block Grade_____ %

2nd Block Grade_____ %

3rd Block Grade_____ %

4th Block Grade_____ %

5th Block Grade_____ %

FINAL GRADE_____ %

....

chapter eleven

Twenty-five Days Later . . . Now What?

J ust because your twenty-five days are up doesn't mean the ride has come to an end. In fact, chances are you're probably enjoying the results you've seen so far and want to jump back in.

But guess what: I'm not going to let you do that—at least not right away.

With any luck, it's taken you only one time through 25Days to forge a new neurological pattern that will, from this point forward, make it easy to keep yourself fit and healthy for life. But if you're not quite there yet, don't worry—you will be.

As you already know, rewiring your brain can take as little as eighteen days, but for most of my clients, twenty-five days has always been the sweet spot. But if that's not your brain, one or two more times around the block (or should I say *blocks*) should do it. Regardless of what stage your brain is at presently in regard to forming a new neurological pattern, you've arrived here because you want to know what's next, so let's get to work!

Remain in the Process

One of the things I'm most known for saying—not just to clients but also to anyone I meet who is looking to improve his or her life—is how important it is to constantly be **"in the process."**

As I wrote in chapter 1, wanting to improve yourself should never be only about losing five pounds in five days, getting skinny for summer, or any other goal that leads to the cram-and-purge methodology that has left you feeling like a failure in the past. The best place you can ever be in life is constantly in the process of getting somewhere. Nothing sounds better than being "in the process" because it's a positive affirmation. And if you're not on the path of working toward a better version of your full potential, then you're in the process of not doing anything.

Being in the process is what kept me going instead of giving up after my three SCAs. Instead of quitting because I couldn't remember what had happened in my life minutes before, I created 25Days to get me through. Staying in the process was what helped me find the motivation to move forward each and every day. It's what eventually led me to share my philosophy and program with my clients. And it's what has allowed me to share 25Days with you.

Why do I say this? Because if you haven't created a new neurological pattern just yet, be patient and put your faith in the program. Even though it may take a few more sessions to reach whatever goals you have for yourself, just being in the process makes you a success every day and brings you even closer to being your best self ever.

So . . . Are You Ready to Start Another 25Days?

Truth be told, there are always a few eager beavers ready to jump right back on board, and if that's you, I admire that spirit. But once you've gotten through 25Days, it's important to take a break for several important reasons:

First, you need time to do some self-reflection of where you were, where you're currently at, and where you want to go next. Because if you don't have some target in mind—if you don't have some goal that always keeps you in the process and moving forward—I guarantee you'll go nowhere fast.

Second, you need time to listen to what your body is trying to tell you and what it needs. If you've done the program right, your body shouldn't be telling you that you need to go back in right away. Your body should be saying "Congratulations! Wonderful job! Feel great about yourself because you stuck it through twenty-five days! Know that you're capable of doing more—and you will soon, I promise—but let's give ourselves a few days to rest."

Third, you need time to give your brain a break. For some people, that can be the hardest thing to do—and maybe that's you. It might be more mentally taxing for you to even think about taking time off because, after all, you just started forging new neurological patterns, and stopping for a short while feels like you're taking three steps back.

But think about this: nobody finishes a week of finals and immediately enrolls in school the next day. Even if you're ambitious enough to take classes over the summer, there's always a period of time off for a reason. That's because even the most prestigious universities and colleges know that it's always healthy to let your brain think in a different direction for a little while.

I get it, though: I've had clients who felt mentally stressed when taking time off 25Days, because of this nagging feeling of "I'm supposed to be somewhere doing something." It's like being on vacation but feeling like you should be at work, even though you don't want to be—because that's what your body and your brain are conditioned to feel.

If that's you, then know this: *All you'll be doing is taking a break for three whole days.*

That's it—just seventy-two hours—a short pause I like to call the **Recover and Discover Three-Day Gateway**. And if you're worried about the damage you can do to your diet in that short amount of time, let me assure you that your brain and body will be just fine. The truth is, once you've been on a structured exercise and nutrition plan like 25Days, you can honestly slide for seventy-two hours. If you jump back on the plan, it's been my experience that none of the damage of eating with calculated liberty really sticks around—nothing. You can actually take a seventy-two-hour hiatus, go back to 25Days, and you really won't pay any penalty at all.

I will say this, though: you have to understand that nutritionally, if you choose to eat junk during those three days, it will play with your insulin levels, and it's going to mess up all of your hormone levels. So if you stray too far from a healthy diet, when you go back into your program, you will genuinely feel less energized. Your body will also say, "Hey! I remember that!" and could go right back to craving certain bad-for-you foods—the same ones you've just beaten using 25Days. That's why it's critical to be smart about how you use those three days. Now let me show you how.

The Recover and Discover Three-Day Gateway

How to Exercise

For all three days, you'll be giving your muscles a break, but I want to be sure your entire body makes the most of those three days. That's why the most intense thing I want you to do is any form of low-intensity activity for a minimum of at least thirty minutes a day, preferably at the same time you typically performed your workouts during the program. If that sounds familiar, it should. Whatever low-impact activity you felt comfortable doing on Secondary Day 3 during the program—whether that was taking a stretching or yoga class or just walking with your dog—that should be the extent of how far you push yourself.

Beyond that, I want you to be good to your body. During this time, the thing to remember is that physically, you should've finished someplace that is exponentially higher than where you started. So reward that effort by getting a massage, going to the spa, seeing a chiropractor, or trying acupuncture. Or just sit in the sauna or just lie out on the beach for three days if that's your thing. The point is, what I want for you in this period is the opportunity to fully recover by doing only activities that are restorative and beneficial to your body. I need you to remain in a state of active healing for the entire three days, doing nothing that may stimulate your central nervous system or prevent your body from fully recovering from the 25Days program.

How to Eat

Like I said earlier in this chapter, the more you abuse this three-day window by eating poorly, the more you can expect to start right back at square one when it comes to cravings. But that doesn't mean the next three days aren't going to please your taste buds.

Go Out as Often as Possible

These three days are a great time to treat yourself by eating out for breakfast, lunch, and dinner. Reason being: you probably avoided many of your favorite restaurants while running through 25Days for the first time—and that's normal. Most people tend to avoid the places they love to eat the most when on a fitness, diet, or lifestyle program.

But I'm not recommending you spoil yourself just for the sake of indulging. I want you to use those meals as a way to test yourself to eat the 25Days way by ordering off menus. Personally, I can eat off of any menu and find either a meal or a combination of individual items to create a breakfast, lunch, or dinner that works within the parameters of the 25Days diet. Now it's your turn—and be ready to be surprised.

What you'll quickly notice is how easy it is. By now, you'll know not just what you're supposed to eat but also what it looks like on your plate. It's time to reward yourself by going to the places you've avoided and challenging yourself to eat within those parameters. Beyond the reward factor, taking this challenge will give you the confidence to know that you can go back to these places that you love once you repeat the 25Days program, giving you even more eating options than you had the first time through.

Go Cook in the Kitchen

Odds are that when you were choosing what to eat for your meals each day, you probably picked certain foods and portions from the charts provided because it was easier. And that's fine, because that's why those charts are there. But as you've noticed, I also provided a variety of recipe options from executive chef Jennifer Jewett, the owner of First Spoonful. That's why another challenge I want you to tackle is to try to cook meals and snacks that are similar in their nutritional balance to what I recommend in 25Days.

If you used some of Jennifer's recipes, you've already done my challenge. But if you haven't, I want you to try to cook a few of them. It's not just about getting you to experience some of the tasty recipes in the book—and trust me when I say they are delicious—but by doing so, I find it inspires my clients to consider their options when at home. It will give you even more confidence when cooking to reshape the meals you may love to make into meals that fit within the 25Days Diet guidelines.

Go Easy on the Snacks

Because you won't be working out during this three-day period (and even if you do something active, it should be a low-intensity activity), your body will naturally be burning fewer calories. That said, if you want to snack between meals, you can. Know that snacks are there for you and you can have them if you want. But just be mindful, based on what you know now. If you don't feel you need to eat them, don't.

Go Nuts on the Last Night!

I love cheesecake, and there's no way you'll ever stop me from eating it at some point in time—and that's fine. It's good to give in every once in a while and actually have your calculated liberty, no matter how nutritionally void or calorie dense it may be. It's great for you physically, due to its effects on ghrelin and leptin, but it's also really great for your mental state. That's why on your third and last day, at dinner, you may have what I call a food parade, or to be more exact, a **One-Hour Absolution**.

That's right. Get ready because you've earned it. And don't worry, because this next meal comes guilt free.

I want you to have a true 100 percent cheat meal that's completely off the reservation. I don't want you to be concerned about what the meal is going to do to your insulin levels. I don't want you to be concerned about what's in it. I don't want you to be concerned about whether you're having a glass of wine or two. I want you to feel like you're having Disneyland on your taste buds: a complete, euphoric dopamine, serotonin, and IGF-I explosion, saved for the last meal of the day.

The only rule: you have one hour to eat wherever you want, whatever you want, and as much as you want. But after that hour is up—you're done.

Most people go too far overboard into the celebration. Instead of going to their favorite restaurant and enjoying a decadent meal for an hour or so, many people use the freedom of a cheat meal as an excuse to cheat with no intention of stopping for hours and hours. They turn a single meal into an ongoing event, starting around happy hour and not ending until midnight.

Within that time, you could consume as much as 10,000 calories (depending on what you're eating), and that is so far off the course of what I'm trying to get your brain and body to do. Limiting you to an hour makes sure you don't take advantage of this free-for-all situation to your detriment. Yes, I'm letting you eat whatever you want, but in a *meal* setting, not a gluttonous feast mode.

If that doesn't make sense, think about this: You wouldn't sit down and eat salad for six hours until midnight, would you? Besides, the fact of the matter is that roughly thirty minutes into your **One-Hour Absolution,** you'll have reset your leptin levels by dropping this presumably carbohydrate-rich calorie bomb on your system. It also means that within thirty minutes, you're technically not hungry anymore, whether you realize it or not. At that point, you're eating just for the sake of eating.

Just remember: this meal is just an opportunity to free your mind, reward yourself for a job well done, and reset your brain around starting the program the very next day when you get back to work. And if you achieve your goals with 25Days, trust me—there will be more of them coming your way, I promise you.

How to Be Aware

I love using the word *awareness* with clients during these three days, because 25Days isn't just about weight loss, working out, and reaching your fitness goals. It's an intention. It's a purposeful thought. It's a conscious decision that you're making because it was a series of unconscious decisions that got you out of shape and into the place you were before 25Days—and still may be in now. But putting things into your conscious mind is going to allow you to continue to succeed.

That said, before you began the program, I asked you to conduct a true evaluation of yourself, and identify and write down five things that you wanted to change, about either yourself or some other aspect of your life. Now it's time to reflect back on those five things and build upon them during these three days of rest.

Like How Far You've Come

I want you to look at the five things you wrote down less than a month ago and see if you can honestly say you've made movement on them. Don't worry if you didn't exactly make all five happen in twenty-five days. I wouldn't have expected you to, and that's not what this is all about. All I want you to do is ask yourself if the needle moved a little further on any of the five. Even if you can say only that you notice an improvement in just one, that's improvement you didn't have twenty-five days ago. So give yourself a big pat on the back and put a big check mark next to it.

Love What You Didn't Expect

Now I want you to put down that list and think about how you feel right now. I'll bet that if you focus hard enough, you'll find a few things different about yourself that you didn't expect. Maybe you've lost your cravings for sugar or soda. Maybe you have more energy or find yourself sleeping more soundly. Maybe you feel stronger, or people have begun noticing a certain confidence in you. Maybe you lost an inch or two around your waist. Whatever they are, I want you to identify the successes you didn't see coming, write them down, and put a check mark next to each one.

Why am I making you place all those check marks? Because there is a constant gratification that comes from realizing you've accomplished something. But even more than that, when you start checking off those first five things, it makes you realize that no matter what you write down—you can accomplish it. That way, if you ever doubt yourself or the program, you'll have five things staring back at you with check marks next to them. Five things you didn't expect to change but did, just by sticking with the program.

But you're not done yet.

Look at Where You Can Go

If you've managed to check off any of those original five things, I want you to write down something new to replace it. So the next time you try the 25Days program, you always have at least five things written down; five things that will allow you to say to yourself, "I'm going to work on this, this, this, this, and this." Because the reality is, once you bring that new thing into awareness, no matter what it is, it's much more likely to get accomplished.

However, this time around, I want you to think beyond the physical. Instead, make it a challenge to look at your mental potential, your emotional potential, your spiritual potential, and your financial potential. I have clients look at a minimum of one thing they'd love to change regarding each of the four. If you like, you could even make them a separate list from your original five. But you'll be amazed at how getting control of the low-hanging fruit—your physical potential—will permeate its way into making you realize that it's possible to, for example, get your finances on track, improve your state of mind, bring happiness to your emotional life, and achieve fulfillment in your spiritual life. It's all about bringing these things into awareness.

Learn from Where You've Been

I want you to put your journal aside and grab your work sheets instead—all of them. I want you to look at each day, each block, and then your final grade. I promised that if you maintained a grade of 85 percent or higher, you'd be sure to achieve your fitness goals. And if you maintained a grade of 85 percent or above, be proud of yourself. But if your grade wasn't 100 percent, then you know there is always room for improvement.

The fact is this: you and only you know that somewhere around, let's say Day 13, you phoned it in—even if you did everything for the day and managed to score 100 percent. Only you know if you gave it your all for each of the twenty-five days or just coasted through them. Even worse, maybe you even fudged your grade a little bit on certain days.

Point being: as you're taking off these three days, hopefully having your tiramisu and hitting the spa, I want you to dig deep and ask yourself, "If I did it again, could I do it better? Could I do it harder? Could I do it more successfully and efficiently? Could I do it with less stress or do it in less time? Could I do it more conveniently? Could I even pull somebody else in to join me on my next 25Days journey?"

There is an unlimited amount of conversations you can have with yourself about how you may be able to do better the next time around. So don't be afraid to ask yourself the hard questions. If you do, you'll find it a lot easier to stick with the program long enough to rewire your brain and establish new neurological patterns a lot faster.

Making the Next 25Days Matter

The beauty of 25Days is that it's ultimately a program that perfects itself continuously. As you adapt to it and become fitter and healthier, the healthy neurological patterns you're creating become stronger and more secure, making it even easier not only to stay the course but also to make 25Days a lifestyle. But because you'll be restarting 25Days in both better physical and neurological shape, it's vital that you make a few slight adjustments to the program to match your current fitness level.

Your Diet

Whether it's your second time around or your seventieth, you won't change the macronutrient balance of each meal and snack, because those formulas are in place to make sure your body has a planned response, which is to utilize fat as energy. It's that macronutrient balance that turns your body into a constant fat-burning machine. Still, there are a few things you can tweak that can yield even better results.

Upgrade What You Eat. Try to think back to what you ate the last time you used 25Days and look at the options you provided yourself. Then ask yourself: "Could I have eaten better versions of those foods?" The way I've organized the food charts, the foods higher up have a lot more to offer, so this time around, try to pick foods slightly above the ones you chose the last time. Or try to find healthier versions of those foods, such as: if you're going to eat chicken, then make it free-range chicken. If you're going to eat a certain vegetable, try to choose an organic, pesticide-free version. You'll be getting the same nutritional benefits, minus any unhealthy chemicals and toxins.

Upgrade Where You Eat. If you're looking for a challenge—one that will leave you feeling even more empowered each time you use 25Days—try eating at a variety of different restaurants. In fact, make a point of eating a different type of cuisine each day, such as Italian, Chinese, Japanese, Mexican, Indian, Thai—you name it. I want you to see how you can eat the 25Days Way anywhere you go, at any restaurant. The more you practice, the more you'll realize you never have to sacrifice in social situations while on the program.

Upgrade the Meals You Make. Look back at your last 25Days experience and count up how many meals you prepared for yourself—not counting any that you made for yourself during your three-day break. If you prepared only a few using the recipes in the book, then make it a goal to add at least one more to that number. If you didn't prepare any, then I want you to prepare at least two—whether it's the recipes in this book or taking a look at other recipes and seeing how you can change the ingredients to match the macronutrient balance expected in each meal and snack.

I know what you're thinking: Why would I tell you to do that if I just insisted you spend three days eating out all over town? If it's possible to eat the 25Days Way in any restaurant, then why not make it easier for myself?

That's because, in reality, there are things we don't know that go into foods when they're being prepared. You may not be entirely aware of what they're being cooked in or what may be added. You don't get to go back into the kitchen and interrogate the chef about whether he's cooking with Himalayan sea salt or regular old iodized table salt. Or if he's using extra-virgin olive oil instead of vegetable oil. The more you experiment with cooking the 25Days Way, the more freedom you'll have at home to create any dish you wish.

Upgrade Your Calendar. Once you've been through 25Days a few times, you're going to notice something. Family barbecues and get-togethers, kids' birthday parties, that company function you have to attend—they all tend to find their way onto the calendar at least a few weeks ahead of time.

Each time you start 25Days, do yourself a favor and grab your calendar, then map it out to see exactly where each day of the plan might fall—particularly your Every-Five-Day Mind Meals. If an event that you know will be a challenge falls directly on a day when you would have a Mind Meal, that might make it a little easier for you, especially because these events tend to have their fair share of starchy carbohydrates such as pasta and potatoes somewhere on the menu.

But if an event that you absolutely can't miss falls a day or two off schedule from your Every-Five-Day Mind Meal, and you think that event might make it difficult for you to stick with the program, don't be afraid to wait a day or so before beginning 25Days again in order to sync it up. Holding off an extra two days won't hurt you, and because your Every-Five-Day Mind Meals come around every five days, that's all you would have to wait—so long as you stick with eating the 25Days Diet for those two days.

Once You've Reached Your Weight Loss Goals

As someone who has been living and teaching the 25Days lifestyle over the last twelve years, I've had to make adjustments to the 25Days Diet for me and my clients once they've hit their fitness goals. And that adjustment is letting you have a One-Hour Absolution every five days.

That's right: I said it. You get to cheat not once a week like most diet programs, but every five days. After the 25Days program changes your neurological patterns and you've reached your weight loss goals, you're free to choose the option to change your Every-Five-Day Mind Meal into a One-Hour Absolution Meal. So instead of my holding you to eating 80 to 120 grams of starchy carbohydrates, you have the freedom to eat what you want, as much as you want, the only limitation being that you get only one hour to do it. However, you're not required to do this, and the best results come from sticking with the Every-Five-Day Mind Meal, so consider your options carefully according to your needs.

That's how people like me and others who have been doing this type of program and staying in shape can live within those parameters and still enjoy the things that they love to eat. Because to make 25Days a lifestyle, it can't be ignored that you're going to crave old-fashioned, high-starch Italian pasta and a piece of cheesecake. And I get that because I do too—but it all has a place. And where that place now exists is where this meal exists, but you have to get to that point to be able to have that freedom every five days.

The only caveat: if you miss any of your workouts during whichever five-day block you're in, or you flubbed any of those days with a score below 85 percent, then stick with the Every-Five-Day Mind Meal at the end of that block.

Your Workouts

The numbers don't lie—but more important, they don't let you fail.

What makes the workouts in 25Days special is their adaptability and their instant feedback. Having not only a grade at the end of each day but also a time that lets you know just how fast or slow you completed your workouts gives you a lot more information than most programs do—information you can use to figure out which portions or days may need a little more attention your next time through the program.

Raise Your Percentages. Before you bother tweaking anything within your workouts, I want you to concentrate on scoring 100 percent each and every day, each and every block, all the way through the program. The grading system does more than help trigger a positive dopamine response at the end of the day. It also keeps you from being too eager to push yourself harder than your body may be able to handle. So if you're not able to get 100 percent, you're honestly not ready to make a change just yet. Your body is still acclimating, so give it the room to adapt.

Raise Your Expectations. Once you've managed to score 100 percent on all twenty-five days in regard to your exercise, you're ready for the next challenge. And what that new challenge may be is entirely up to you. Since most people start 25Days as a beginner, the plan for you could be to try it again as an intermediate exerciser. Maybe the best plan for you is to stick with the same level as before, but this time you'll try to score 100 percent every day *and* do each workout a little faster.

Or you could stick with the same level and try to match your workout times but make a point of trying a harder version of one or two exercises in the program. You can raise your repetitions, lower your rest times in between, add an extra round, or even reverse the order of the exercises. Any one of these tweaks is more than enough to change the program, so it's not like you need to do them all. No matter how many changes you implement, even if just one, you'll be progressing enough in the program to keep your body and mind challenged the entire time.

Raise Your Resistance. Even though many of the exercises in 25Days require nothing more than your body weight as resistance, you're free to add other pieces of equipment—such as dumbbells, exercise bands, weighted vests, and other fitness tools—to customize your workout according to their ability. The simple act of holding a pair of dumbbells in your hands during many of the moves that leave your hands free will make the exercises that much harder to do.

Raise Your Awareness. Instead of timing your entire workout from start to finish, if you don't mind micromanaging, try timing each round as well. That way, you can see how well you're improving with each round on every day, which may give you more insight into where you may be putting more effort into certain portions of your workout.

Once You've Reached Your Fitness Goals

With exercise, there is always the ability (if you remain healthy) to become stronger and faster—so how will you know when to stop?

Somewhere way down the road, once you've climbed the workout ladder to the point where you're able to perform the most advanced versions of the exercises in the book with the least amount of rest and the greatest number of reps—you'll find yourself looking for the next way to see progress. That's when I'll have you change the structure of your workout.

Instead of alternating between Primary Day A and Primary Day B every other day, I want you to start doing both Primary Days back to back, followed by a Secondary Day—then repeat. So instead of following this type of exercise schedule (**A**1**B**2**A**3**B**1, and so on), you'll now try **AB**1**AB**2**AB**3, and so on. This will have you doing three or four strength-training workouts each block, instead of just two or three.

But know this: everyone's body is different. And only you will know what's best for you. If you're entirely fine using the original version of the workout, and you're happy with the results you've seen from it, I won't discourage you from continuing to use it. But don't be afraid to explore and see what that new physique of yours is capable of. I guarantee you: it won't let you down.

Keep a Journal

There's a story I often use to get clients to understand the theory behind living to one's full potential. A woman finds herself in Heaven and asks God who is the most successful woman in all of humankind. God looks around, then points to a random person in the crowd. The woman turns to God and says, "You must be mistaken. I knew her on Earth, and she wasn't very successful." And God simply nods and says, "I know, but she could have been. She just never lived up to her full potential."

The question I have for you is this: *Are you the best version of yourself that you can be?*

As you go through 25Days once more—and every time you use it—I want you to ask yourself, "Am I living up to my full potential?" Then I want you to think about what your "full potential" looks like, feels like, walks like, and talks like. I want you to focus on what your full potential is, because everyone's is different.

Whenever you see athletes or celebrities at the top of their game, it's only natural to feel that they're living up to their full potential—but how do you know? You don't. You have no idea if they could've achieved more and just lack the mental wherewithal or motivation to go any further.

So before you have a meal or snack or begin your workout, ask yourself if you're living up to your full potential. Just getting yourself to address that subject before you eat or exercise can be a last-minute motivator that can help you achieve a higher score at that moment. After you've eaten or exercised, I want you to ask yourself again: "Am I living up to my full potential? Am I the best version of myself that I can be?"

Once You've Reached Your Personal Goals

Remember what I said about staying in the process? That if you're not in the process of working toward a better version of yourself, then you're in the process of not doing anything? I want you to keep journaling. Long after you've formed the neurological patterns that will help you stay fit, healthy, and lean for life. Long after you've reached your goals and continue to use the process. Long after all of it.

I never want you to forget how far you came; but, more important, I want you to realize that the person you've become—that best possible version of yourself—can make an impact on bringing out the best possible version of someone else.

Look outside your physical self and ask yourself, "How did doing

25Days cause me to start acting differently in other areas of my life, such as at work, at home, in the relationships I have with my friends?" And so on. And if you're happy with those results, as I know you will be, then ask yourself, "Was I able to inspire others to do more with their lives because I expected more out of myself—or did I just keep it all to myself?"

There is no harm in keeping it all to yourself. But the real value when you succeed with 25Days (and prove what's possible by changing how your brain works) is how you're able to inspire, talk to, or encourage others to follow along with you. By inspiring others and leading the way, by trying to empower them and take them with you on the journey, you'll enjoy the greatest feeling of success you'll ever experience with 25Days. And I know: because you've allowed me to take you on that journey.

I'll see you—in twenty-five days.

Acknowledgments

In order to properly give appreciation to those who set me on the path to end up where I am today, I have to start near the beginning: being sixteen years old and having Arnold Schwarzenegger come to my high school advanced PE class and telling me to my face, "You can do *anything* you want to do, and everything you want lies behind the discipline in staying fit and getting strong! Never stop being healthy, and never stop helping your friends and family to become healthy." A big thank-you to the Terminator for being the first to inspire me down the path of becoming a trainer in the fall of 1990.

To the many clients and friends who would come after the fateful day of October 4, 2004—who I would eventually use as "test subjects" for what eventually became 25Days—you knew a different version of me than everyone had before. Thank you for your patience and trust. Kata Rhe, I am eternally indebted and grateful. Dr. Dawood Darbar and the brilliant nurses and staff of the Vanderbilt University Page-Campbell Heart Institute who saved my life, you can never realize the roles you played. Thank you. And to Dr. Sumeet Chugh and the Cedars-Sinai Heart Institute, thank you for keeping me healthy and on the cutting edge of the science of understanding sudden cardiac arrest.

To the many actors, musicians, models, athletes, and entertainment clients I have been blessed to work with (even for short periods), I can honestly say I have had nothing but wonderful experiences with you and am thankful for you all to have been a part of my journey: Nazr Mohammed, Tom Green, Rick Brothers, Boris Kodjoe, Lance Bass, Keith Urban, Florida

Georgia Line—Tyler Hubbard and Brian Kelley (and their lovely wives)—Bruno Gunn, Rick Cosnett, Jesse L. Martin, and many, many more, you are all some of the best people I know in any walk of life. Thank you.

To my executive producers of STRONG, Dave Broome and Sylvester Stallone, thank you for giving me an opportunity to take my militant training mind and style to network TV! To Gunter Schlierkamp and Kim Lyons: you guys are my family in the industry and life; you have inspired me, encouraged, laughed, and cried, and stuck by me for over a decade—endless thanks. Robert Cabral—the second coolest guy on the planet; you've always had my back—thank you for staying true.

To all the team that made this book possible and believed in my dream—my mad scientist writer, buddy, and collaborator, Myatt Murphy—you are *the* man! My literary agent, Heather Jackson—if I had a team of people like you, I would run for president . . . and win! The amazing staff and editors at Simon & Schuster, Diana Ventimiglia, Michele Martin, Cindy Ratzlaff: thank you all for taking a chance and making this process exciting and such a wonderful experience—here's to many more! Jennifer Jewett and the team at First Spoonful Meals for creating some of the most amazing healthy recipes that have ever been put into print. Photographer Teren Oddo, MUA Tara Bre, and impromptu fitness model Patti Panucci, thank you guys so much for pulling off the impossible shoot in record time! To my publicists, Tanya Taylor, Carrie Simons, Ashley Sandberg, and the rest of the team at Triple7 PR, you girls are amazing; thank you for kicking down doors for me. My talent agent at WME, Evan Warner, thank you for bringing me to STRONG and opening the doors for everything. And a very special thank-you to my dear friend, client, manager, super cheerleader, and the best connector in the business, Carey Nelson Burch—I would literally have nothing if it weren't for the connections, introductions, and indirect relationships you have created for me.

To my family and close friends, you have been there the whole way and have watched it all unfold. I appreciate you more than you will ever know, and I hope we have many more memories to share. Uncle Gary: thank you for always inspiring me to think deeply and question everything, and for inspiring my early love of sports by yelling at the TV during the Kentucky basketball games. Aunt Linda: thank you for inspiring me to always remember to remain active by watching you doing a constant array of workouts, aerobics, tennis, swimming, or anything fitness related when I was a kid! Amy, Matt, and Steve . . . you guys were the best "home team" to have grown up with. My cousins, Ashley, Steve, and Allie, so proud of you all and the wonderful adults you have become and the happy and healthy families you are creating. Doug Blake: thank you for fostering my love of baseball, rock & roll, sarcasm, and fast muscle cars. Dr. Vera Dunn: thank you for showing me a deep compassion and leadership in unpacking my overly ambitious and cluttered mind. I am not sure I could have accomplished any of this without you.

Last, and most important, my parents. You two have been on every journey, every ride, every scrape and bruise (*figuratively and literally*) with me since I began. Thank you for putting me into sports at age four and for teaching me the value of resilience, determination, character, and honesty. Thank you for pushing me, trusting me, praying for me, and paying that ridiculous grocery bill when I was a teenager determined to work out five hours a day. Mom, thank you for teaching me good manners, the gift of endless conversation with strangers, the importance of reading books, and a broad vocabulary. Dad, thank you for being my first and longest-living hero—teaching me intensity, focus, a ridiculous work ethic, and that I can do anything if I want it bad enough and can think it through. Thank you both for your undying love and support. I could have done nothing in my life without you. I love you.

Index

addiction, 52
adenosine triphosphate (ATP), 122, 125
adrenaline, 139
aerobic energy pathway/metabolism, 123
aging process, accelerating, 53
alcohol, as no-no, 42, 50–52
Almond Butter Dipping Sauce, 107
almonds, 17
  Almond Milk, 81
  Toasted Almond Pesto, 83–84
Alternating Donkey Kicks, 187–88
Alternating Supermans, 163–64
Alzheimer's disease, 53
amino acids, 18, 43
anabolic synthesis state, 36, 39
anaerobic energy pathway, 123, 124
anticipation, 139
apples, 42, 55, 67
artificial sweeteners, 45–49
aspartame, 45, 46
ATP-CP system, 122
avocados, 17, 48
  Pea and Edamame Hummus, 109
awareness, 248–50, 255
  body awareness, 121
  of how far you've come, 248
  of what you didn't expect, 248–49

of where you can go, 249
of where you've been, 250

balance, 18
beans, 44
beef, 17
Beets, Pickled, 98–99
Big Bicycles, 165–66
biological values (BV), 59
bison: Braised Bison–Stuffed Cabbage
  Rolls with Sweet-and-Sour Tomato
  Sauce, 103–4
bloating, 40, 46
blood pressure, 52
blood sugar cravings, 32
blood sugar levels, 44, 47, 51, 54
brain:
  and dopamine, 9–11
  and exercise, 120–21
  rewiring, 6–8
brain barrier:
  breaking, 9–14
  daily grade, 12
  and 85 percent promise, 13–14
  figuring your scores, 11
  Put-Ins, 11
Braised Bison–Stuffed Cabbage Rolls
  with Sweet-and-Sour Tomato Sauce,
  103–4
bread, 44, 70, 71